Research on Mycotoxins - From Mycotoxigenic Fungi to Innovative Strategies of Diagnosis, Control and Detoxification

Edited by Mehdi Razzaghi-Abyaneh, Masoomeh Shams-Ghahfarokhi and Mahendra Rai

Published in London, United Kingdom

Research on Mycotoxins - From Mycotoxigenic Fungi to Innovative Strategies of Diagnosis, Control and Detoxification
http://dx.doi.org/10.5772/intechopen.1003511
Edited by Mehdi Razzaghi-Abyaneh, Masoomeh Shams-Ghahfarokhi and Mahendra Rai

Contributors
Ahmet Düzel, Archana Keche, Ebrahim Molaee-aghaee, Fabrice De Paul Tatfo Keutchatang, Girish Patil, Isabelle Sandrine Bouelet Ntsama, Jiang Li, Leila Faeli, Madhavi Madkey, Mehdi Fathollahi, Parisa Shavali-gilani, Paul Richard Keutchatang, Preeti Kaur, Razieh Noroozi, Shubhankar Anand, Xiangfeng Zheng, Zhenquan Yang, Zhongyang Cao

First published in London, United Kingdom, 2025 by IntechOpen
IntechOpen is the global imprint of INTECHOPEN LIMITED, registered in England and Wales, registration number: 11086078, 167-169 Great Portland Street, London, W1W 5PF, United Kingdom

For EU product safety concerns: IN TECH d.o.o., Prolaz Marije Krucifikse Kozulić 3, 51000 Rijeka, Croatia, info@intechopen.com or visit our website at intechopen.com.

British Library Cataloguing-in-Publication Data
A catalogue record for this book is available from the British Library

Research on Mycotoxins - From Mycotoxigenic Fungi to Innovative Strategies of Diagnosis, Control and Detoxification
Edited by Mehdi Razzaghi-Abyaneh, Masoomeh Shams-Ghahfarokhi and Mahendra Rai
p. cm.
Print ISBN 978-1-83634-110-9
Online ISBN 978-1-83634-109-3
eBook (PDF) ISBN 978-1-83634-111-6

Meet the editors

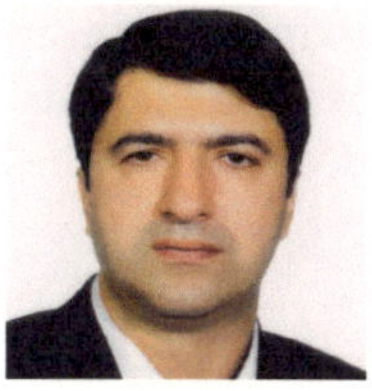

Professor Mehdi Razzaghi-Abyaneh was born in Tehran, Iran. He obtained his Ph.D. degree in Medical Mycology from Tarbiat Modares University in Tehran, Iran. Dr. Razzaghi-Abyaneh pursued a 12-month sabbatical on the identification of antifungal compounds from bioactive plants at the Graduate School of Agriculture, Tokyo University, in the Laboratory of Applied Biological Chemistry from 2006 to 2007. He is currently a full professor and eminent research scientist at the Pasteur Institute of Iran (Tehran, Iran), where he is working on mycotoxins and mycotoxigenic fungi as well as antifungal nanomaterial and biologically active antifungals of plant, fungal and bacterial origin for more than 25 years. He has supervised and been the advisor of several Ph.D. and MSc theses. Dr. Razzaghi-Abyaneh has published over 180 papers in peer-reviewed international journals, 12 books, and a number of book chapters. His research is focused on the chemical basis of plant-fungal interactions and determining the mode of action of antifungal bioactive compounds of natural origin as small and macromolecules at cellular and molecular levels.

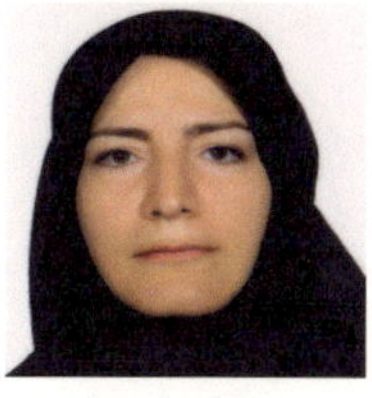

Professor Masoomeh Shams-Ghahfarokhi is working as a faculty member at Tarbiat Modares University in Tehran, Iran, where she has worked for around 25 years. After graduating in Medical Mycology in 2000, Dr. Shams-Ghahfarokhi passed a training course as a JSPS fellow in Japan during 2005-2007. Her investigation focuses on identifying and isolating antifungal compounds from natural resources (including plants and organisms) and their molecular aspects on the activity of pathogenic fungi. She actively evaluates the inhibitory effects of bio-nanomaterials and anti-scaling membranes for the selective treatment of fungal infections and their mechanism of action on the cellular and molecular levels. She is also investigating the identification of pathogenic fungi and their genetic diversity by using molecular techniques such as Sequencing, Real time-PCR, Multiplex-PCR, etc. Dr Shams-Ghahfarokhi has around two decades of teaching and research experience, and she has been a supervisor and advisor for many M. Sc. and Ph.D. theses.

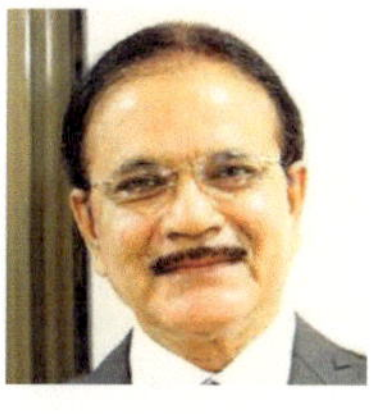

Professor Mahendra Rai is a visiting scientist at Nicolaus Copernicus University in Torun, Poland. He published over 450 research papers, over 100 popular articles in Indian and foreign journals, and 75 books from reputed publishers like Elsevier, Springer, CRC, Taylor and Francis, Wiley, and Scientific Publisher. He is a member of several scientific societies and has been a national scholar for five years. He received several prestigious awards, including the Father T. A. Mathias Award (1989) from the All India Association for Christian Higher Education and the Medini Award (1999) from the Department of Environment and Forest, Government of India. He also received a SERC visiting fellowship from the Department of Science and Technology (1996), an INSA visiting fellowship by the Indian National Science Academy (1998), and a TWAS-UNESCO Associateship (2002) in Italy. Dr. Rai was also awarded a University Grants Commission-Basic Scientific Research (UGC-BSR) faculty fellowship by the University Grants Commission, New Delhi (2017-2020) and an NAWA (Polish National Agency for Academic Exchange) fellowship by the Polish Government (2021-2023). He serves as a referee for 20 international journals and is a member of the editorial board of 10 national and international journals. He has approximately three decades of teaching and research experience. His research mainly focuses on plant and nano-based bioactive compounds against human pathogenic microbes.

Contents

Preface IX

Chapter 1 1
From Fungi to Food Safety: Advancing Mycotoxin Research and Solutions
by Preeti Kaur and Shubhankar Anand

Chapter 2 23
Detection and Detoxification Methods for Mycotoxins: From Classical to New Trends
by Ahmet Düzel

Chapter 3 37
Mycotoxins Diagnostic Methods from Past to Present
by Leila Faeli

Chapter 4 53
Mycotoxins and Mitigation Plan
by Mehdi Fathollahi, Razieh Noroozi, Parisa Shavali-gilani and Ebrahim Molaee-aghaee

Chapter 5 71
Research Progress on Prevention and Elimination of Patulin in Food
by Xiangfeng Zheng, Zhongyang Cao, Jiang Li and Zhenquan Yang

Chapter 6 89
Mycotoxicoses in Humans
by Girish Patil, Archana Keche and Madhavi Madkey

Chapter 7 103
Mycotoxins in Chicken Farming: What You Need to Know
by Fabrice De Paul Tatfo Keutchatang, Isabelle Sandrine Bouelet Ntsama and Paul Richard Keutchatang

Preface

Mycotoxins are a group of fungal secondary metabolites primarily produced by fungi from the genera *Aspergillus, Penicillium, and Fusarium*. Contamination of food, animal feed, and agricultural crops by various mycotoxins poses a significant risk of intoxication to humans and animals while also causing substantial economic losses on a global scale. In addition to their mutagenic and carcinogenic effects on humans, it is estimated that the annual losses due to three major mycotoxins, aflatoxin, fumonisin, and deoxynivalenol, reach as high as 1.2 billion USD, impacting maize, groundnut, and wheat growers worldwide.

In a global context, mycotoxin contamination is a major concern for third-world countries and developed countries in Europe and America. Pertaining to the ongoing complications arising from mycotoxin contamination of human and animal foods all over the world, research on different aspects of mycotoxins with a special focus on diagnosis, control and detoxification approaches has received major consideration as one of the most exciting disciplines of medicine to agriculture research. Nowadays, mycotoxin research has been expanded beyond the traditional approaches to modern strategies for pre- and post-harvest management of mycotoxin contamination of agricultural commodities.

The book, comprising seven chapters, covers some important aspects of mycotoxin contamination of food and agricultural crops, from diagnostic methods to mitigation plans for control of mycotoxin contamination, detoxification of mycotoxins by novel approaches and finally, the importance of mycotoxins in human and animal health.

We sincerely appreciate the valuable contributions of all the authors who played a crucial role in achieving the goals of this book. Our gratitude also extends to the IntechOpen publishing team, particularly Kristina Kardum Cvitan, for her dedicated assistance in coordinating the book and scheduling our activities.

Mehdi Razzaghi-Abyaneh
Department of Mycology,
Pasteur Institute of Iran,
Tehran, Iran

Masoomeh Shams-Ghahfarokhi
Department of Mycology,
Faculty of Medical Sciences,
Tarbiat Modares University,
Tehran, Iran

Mahendra Rai
Department of Microbiology,
Nicolaus Copernicus University,
Torun, Poland

Chapter 1

From Fungi to Food Safety: Advancing Mycotoxin Research and Solutions

Preeti Kaur and Shubhankar Anand

Abstract

This chapter delves into the dynamic field of mycotoxin research and the creative approaches being used to improve food safety by addressing the problems caused by mycotoxigenic fungus. Toxic secondary metabolites pose a serious danger to human health and food security. They are produced by fungi including *Aspergillus*, *Penicillium*, and *Fusarium* species. Because of their prevalence in crops, particularly staple grains like peanuts, wheat, and maize, much study is required to comprehend their methods of development and create practical mitigation measures. Mycotoxin production in fungus is influenced by genetic and metabolic processes that have been clarified by recent advances in mycotoxin research. Designing focused strategies to stop fungal contamination in agricultural contexts requires careful consideration of these observations. Innovative strategies include the creation of biocontrol agents, genetic engineering of crops to increase resistance, and environmentally friendly detoxifying techniques to reduce mycotoxin contamination in food and feed. Additionally, advancements in analytical methods including Mass Spectrometry (MS), biosensors, and High-Performance Liquid Chromatography (HPLC) have transformed the identification and measurement of mycotoxins in a variety of matrices. These delicate techniques are essential for adhering to regulations and guaranteeing that food safety requirements are fulfilled. This chapter also outlines new directions in mycotoxin research, including the effects of global commerce on the regional distribution of mycotoxin contamination and the dynamics of fungal growth and mycotoxin production.

Keywords: mycotoxin, detoxification, genetic engineering, mass spectrometry, high-performance liquid chromatography

1. Introduction

Fungi are found everywhere and have both positive and negative effects on human society [1, 2]. While they play important roles in processes like decomposition and food production, they can also produce mycotoxins, which are harmful to human and animal health [3]. Mycotoxins are toxic substances naturally produced by certain fungi, and their presence in crops can have serious health effects [4]. They are a leading cause of foodborne illnesses, economic losses in agriculture, and regulatory challenges [5]. Fungi, which include molds, yeasts, and mushrooms, have had a significant impact on human history. While some fungi are beneficial, others pose threats to food security and human health. Mycotoxins are among the most concerning threats, as they are toxic fungal byproducts that can contaminate various food crops, leading to severe health consequences and economic losses worldwide [6]. Mycotoxins are a complex challenge at the intersection of agriculture, food safety, and public health [7]. Their presence in the food supply has been a longstanding issue, and it is important to develop comprehensive strategies to mitigate their impact. The global nature of food production and trade, along with the effects of climate change on fungal growth and toxin levels, has intensified the urgency of addressing mycotoxin contamination [8]. The most dangerous mycotoxins include aflatoxins, ochratoxins, trichothecenes, fumonisins, zearalenone, and deoxynivalenol (DON) [9, 10]. These toxins are produced by certain species of *Aspergillus*, *Penicillium*, *Trichoderma*, and *Fusarium*, and commonly contaminate staple crops such as wheat, maize, peanuts, and coffee [6]. Each mycotoxin has distinct biological effects, with some being acutely toxic, while others are carcinogenic or immunosuppressive. For example, Aflatoxin B1 is a highly potent natural carcinogen that can cause liver cancer in humans [11]. Fumonisin B1 is associated with esophageal cancer and birth defects, particularly in regions where maize is a dietary staple [12]. The global impact of mycotoxin contamination is significant. The Food and Agriculture Organization (FAO) estimates that mycotoxins affect as much as 25% of global food crops annually, leading to direct losses in food quality and quantity, economic consequences, increased healthcare costs, and reduced productivity, especially in developing countries [13].

Dealing with mycotoxins is challenging due to their chemical diversity and ability to contaminate a wide range of foods under various environmental conditions [14]. These toxins are stable and difficult to remove once they have contaminated food products. Factors such as warm temperatures and high humidity, which are becoming more prevalent due to climate change, can lead to increased mycotoxin production [15]. Addressing the mycotoxin problem requires a multifaceted approach involving prevention, detection, and mitigation [16]. Prevention efforts should focus on improving agricultural practices, including crop rotation, the use of resistant crop varieties, and better storage techniques. Advances in biotechnology, such as genetically modified crops with enhanced resistance to fungal infection, also show promise in reducing mycotoxin contamination [17]. Detection and monitoring are critical components of any mycotoxin management strategy. While traditional methods like Thin-Layer Chromatography (TLC) and Enzyme-Linked Immunosorbent Assay (ELISA) have been widely used, recent advancements in analytical technologies, such as Liquid Chromatography-Mass Spectrometry (LC-MS), offer improved accuracy and efficiency in detecting mycotoxins [18]. In addition to traditional and advanced analytical methods, rapid detection technologies are being developed to provide real-time monitoring of mycotoxin levels [19]. Biosensors, for example, offer highly sensitive and specific detection of mycotoxins, particularly in regions with limited access to laboratory facilities [20].

Mitigation strategies for mycotoxin contamination vary depending on the type of mycotoxin and the food involved [14]. Physical methods like sorting, cleaning, and heat treatment can reduce mycotoxin levels in some cases. Chemical detoxification methods and biological control methods, such as the use of non-toxigenic fungal strains, also show promise in reducing mycotoxin contamination [21]. The regulation of mycotoxins is intricate and varies significantly across different regions. International organizations like the Codex Alimentarius Commission (CAC) have established guidelines and maximum permissible limits for certain mycotoxins in food and feed [22]. These guidelines serve as a reference for national regulatory bodies, which may set their own standards based on local risk assessments and dietary patterns. However, achieving global harmonization of mycotoxin regulations remains a challenge, especially in international trade, where differing standards can lead to trade disputes and barriers [23]. Looking ahead, ongoing research and innovation will be crucial in advancing our understanding of mycotoxins and developing effective solutions to mitigate their impact. Emerging technologies, such as next-generation sequencing (NGS) and omics approaches, are providing new insights into the genetic and environmental factors that influence mycotoxin production [24]. These technologies have the potential to identify new targets for intervention, whether through the development of resistant crop varieties, the application of precision agriculture techniques, or the design of novel detoxification strategies. Climate change presents both challenges and opportunities for mycotoxin management [25, 26]. Changing environmental conditions may lead to shifts in the prevalence and distribution of mycotoxins, making it more difficult to predict and manage contamination events [27]. However, increased awareness of the links between climate change and food safety may drive investment in research and the development of more resilient agricultural systems [28]. Ultimately, the goal of mycotoxin research and management is to ensure that food systems are safe, sustainable, and resilient in the face of these challenges [29]. This will require a collaborative effort involving scientists, policymakers, industry stakeholders, and consumers [30]. By advancing our understanding of fungi and their toxins, and by developing and implementing effective solutions, we can work toward a future where mycotoxins no longer threaten global food safety and public health [31].

This chapter explores mycotoxins in detail, including the types produced by fungi, their impact on food safety, and the latest advancements in mycotoxin research. It also discusses strategies being developed to reduce mycotoxin contamination and ensure safer food supplies worldwide. In this context, the journey from fungi to food safety is not just a scientific endeavor but a critical component of ensuring the well-being of populations around the world. As we continue to explore the complexities of mycotoxin contamination and develop innovative approaches to combat it, we move closer to achieving a safer, healthier, and more secure food supply for all.

2. Types and origins of mycotoxins

Mycotoxins are toxic compounds produced as secondary metabolites by various fungi, particularly by *Aspergillus* [32], *Fusarium* [33], and *Penicillium* species [34]. These fungi can colonize crops such as cereals, nuts, fruits, and spices, especially under conditions of high humidity and temperature, leading to the production of mycotoxins. The most well-known and studied mycotoxins include aflatoxins [35], ochratoxins [36], fumonisins [37], zearalenone [38], and deoxynivalenol (DON) [39].

2.1 Aflatoxins

Aflatoxins, one of the most poisonous mycotoxins, are primarily produced by *Aspergillus flavus* [40] and *Aspergillus parasiticus* [41]. They predominantly grow in crops like cereals, nuts, legumes, and dried foods like herbs and spices. Aflatoxins are carcinogenic, with aflatoxin B1 being the most toxic and well-documented for its ability to cause liver cancer in humans and animals [42]. Aflatoxins in food products pose a major threat to public health, particularly in regions with inadequate food storage and processing practices [43].

2.2 Ochratoxins

Ochratoxins, produced by species like *Aspergillus ochraceus* [44] and *Penicillium verrucosum* [45, 46], are primarily found in cereals, coffee, and dried fruits [47]. Ochratoxin A (OTA) is the most toxic variant, known for its nephrotoxic effects, potentially leading to kidney damage and cancer [48]. The ability of ochratoxins to withstand food processing methods such as baking and roasting further complicates efforts to mitigate their presence in the food chain [49].

2.3 Fumonisins

Fumonisins are commonly found in maize and maize-based products and produced by *Fusarium* species [50]. Fumonisin B1, the most common of this group, has been linked to esophageal cancer and neural tube defects in humans, as well as leukoencephalomalacia in horses [51]. The prevalence of fumonisins in staple foods like maize makes them a significant food safety issue, particularly in regions where maize is a dietary staple [12].

2.4 Zearalenone

Zearalenone is the second most predominant mycotoxin produced by *Fusarium* species, known for its estrogenic effects [52]. It can contaminate cereals such as wheat, oats, maize, and barley [53]. The estrogenic properties of zearalenone can lead to reproductive disorders in livestock, making it a concern for both food and feed safety [54].

2.5 Deoxynivalenol (DON)

Also known as vomitoxin, deoxynivalenol is produced by *Fusarium graminearum* and is commonly found in cereals such as wheat, barley, and oats [55, 56]. DON is

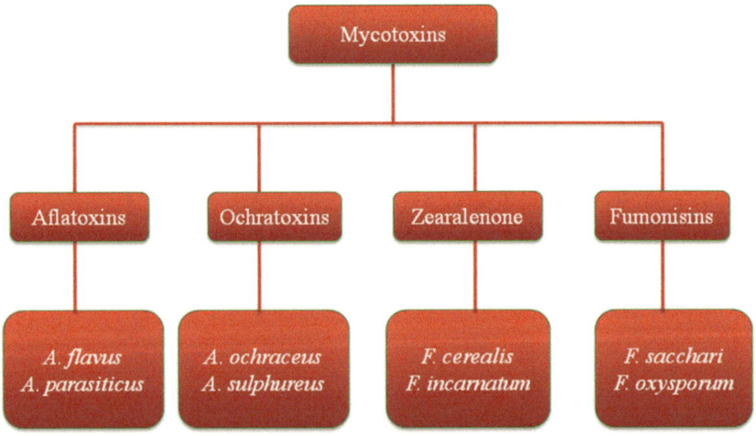

Figure 1.
Different mycotoxins and their causative microorganism.

known to cause gastrointestinal distress and immune suppression in animals, and its presence in food products can lead to significant economic losses due to its impact on livestock health and productivity [57]. **Figure 1** shows different mycotoxins and their source.

3. Causes and consequences of mycotoxin contamination

3.1 Environmental factors

Mycotoxin production is influenced by various environmental factors, such as temperature, humidity, and the presence of pests [58]. Warm and humid conditions promote fungal growth and mycotoxin production, which can occur during crop growth in the field or in storage facilities [59]. The geographic location of crop production also affects the risk of mycotoxin contamination, with tropical and subtropical regions being particularly vulnerable [25].

3.2 Agricultural practices

Certain agricultural practices can increase the risk of mycotoxin contamination [60]. For instance, monocropping, which involves growing the same crop repeatedly on the same land, can cause a buildup of fungal spores in the soil, raising the likelihood of contamination [61]. Improper irrigation practices and the use of contaminated seeds can also contribute to fungal colonization and mycotoxin production [62, 63].

3.3 Post-harvest handling and storage

Post-harvest handling and storage conditions play a crucial role in determining the extent of mycotoxin contamination [64]. Poor storage conditions, such as inadequate drying of crops before storage or the presence of pests, can create an environment favorable for fungal growth and mycotoxin production [58]. The duration of storage also impacts the risk of mycotoxin accumulation, with longer storage periods posing higher risks [65].

3.4 Economic impact

Mycotoxin contamination has significant economic implications. Contaminated crops may be unfit for human consumption or animal feed, resulting in direct financial losses for farmers [66]. Additionally, mycotoxin contamination can lead to trade restrictions and the rejection of export shipments, further worsening economic losses [67]. The costs associated with implementing mycotoxin control measures, such as testing and remediation, also contribute to the economic burden [68].

3.5 Health consequences

The health consequences of mycotoxin exposure can be severe. Chronic exposure to low levels of mycotoxins, such as aflatoxins, can cause liver cancer, immune suppression, and stunted growth in children [69]. Acute exposure to high levels of mycotoxins can lead to immediate health effects, including vomiting, diarrhea, and in extreme cases, death. The impact of mycotoxins on public health is particularly significant in developing countries, where food safety regulations and monitoring systems may be less stringent [70].

4. Advancements in mycotoxin detection and monitoring

Effective mycotoxin management begins with accurate detection and monitoring. Over time, significant progress has been made in developing analytical methods for detecting mycotoxins in food and feed. **Figure 2** represents the different methods of detection of mycotoxins.

4.1 Traditional methods of analysis

Historically, mycotoxin detection has relied on traditional methods such as thin-layer chromatography (TLC) and enzyme-linked immunosorbent assay (ELISA) [71]. While these methods are still widely used due to their simplicity and cost-effectiveness, they have limitations in terms of sensitivity, specificity, and the ability to detect multiple mycotoxins simultaneously.

4.2 High-performance liquid chromatography (HPLC)

High-performance liquid chromatography (HPLC) has become the most reliable method for determining mycotoxins due to its high sensitivity and accuracy [72]. When coupled with mass spectrometry (MS), HPLC can detect and quantify multiple mycotoxins in a single run, making it a powerful tool for comprehensive mycotoxin analysis [73]. The advanced form of HPLC technology, called

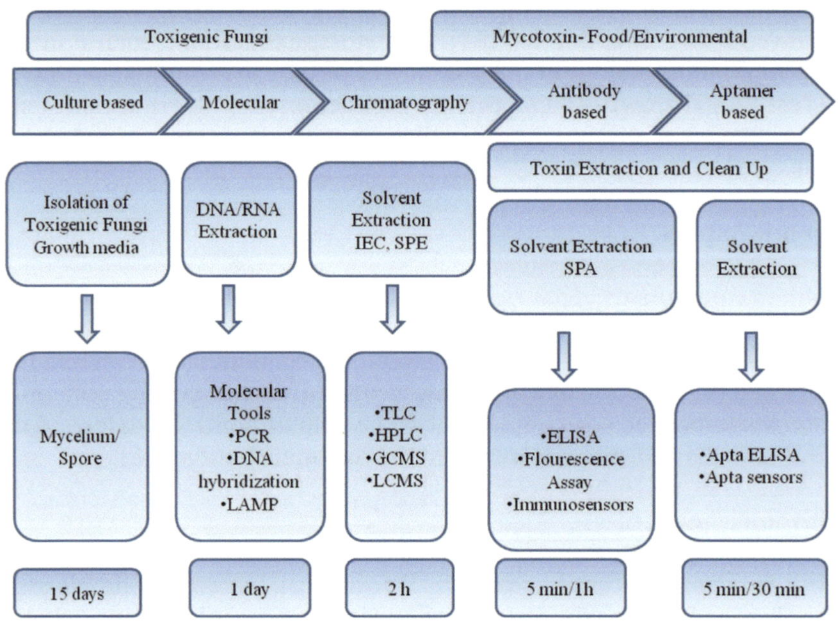

Figure 2.
Methods of detection of mycotoxins.

ultra-high-performance liquid chromatography (UHPLC), offers even greater speed and resolution [74].

4.3 Rapid detection methods

Recent years have seen the development of rapid detection methods that offer faster and more convenient mycotoxin analysis. For example, Lateral flow immunoassays (LFIA) provide a quick and easy-to-use solution for on-site testing, allowing for real-time monitoring of mycotoxin levels [75]. These methods are particularly useful in scenarios where quick decision-making is required, such as during harvest or in storage facilities [76].

4.4 Biosensors

Biosensors represent a cutting-edge approach to mycotoxin detection. These devices use biological recognition elements, such as antibodies or enzymes, to detect the presence of mycotoxins [20]. The interaction between the mycotoxin and the recognition element generates a signal that can be measured and correlated to mycotoxin concentration [77]. Biosensors offer the potential for highly sensitive, specific, and rapid mycotoxin detection, making them an attractive option for future mycotoxin monitoring efforts [75, 78].

4.5 Next-generation sequencing (NGS)

Next-generation sequencing (NGS) or advanced high-throughput sequencing is a modern tool for identifying the fungal communities associated with mycotoxin production [24]. By sequencing the DNA of fungi present in crops, researchers can identify the specific species responsible for mycotoxin production and monitor changes in fungal populations over time [79]. NGS can also provide insights into the genetic factors that regulate mycotoxin biosynthesis, opening up new avenues for targeted interventions [80].

5. Strategies for mycotoxin mitigation

Mycotoxin contamination poses significant risks to food and feed safety. **Table 1** represents the different strategies for mycotoxin control. To mitigate this risk, several strategies have been developed, as shown in **Figure 3**.

5.1 Pre-harvest interventions

Pre-harvest interventions aim to reduce the risk of field contamination by mycotoxins [81]. Strategies include promoting resistant crop varieties, crop rotation, and using biocontrol agents such as non-toxigenic strains of *Aspergillus* to reduce aflatoxin contamination in crops like corn and peanuts [82].

5.2 Good agricultural practices (GAP)

Good agricultural practices encompass techniques to minimize mycotoxin contamination during crop production [83]. This includes proper irrigation management,

Category	Control strategy	Description
Pre-harvest	Crop rotation	Regularly changing the type of crop grown in a field to reduce the buildup of mycotoxin-producing fungi.
	Resistant crop varieties	Breeding or using genetically modified crops resistant to mycotoxin-producing fungal species.
	Fungicide application	Applying chemicals to reduce fungal infections on crops, particularly during critical growth stages.
	Irrigation management	Ensuring optimal water supply to avoid plant stress, which makes crops more susceptible to mycotoxins.
	Pest control	Managing insect vectors that can wound plants and promote fungal infections.
Post-harvest	Proper drying	Drying crops immediately after harvest to moisture levels below 13% to inhibit fungal growth.
	Temperature control	Storing crops at low temperatures to reduce fungal growth and mycotoxin production.
	Controlled atmosphere storage	Reducing oxygen levels or adjusting gas mixtures to inhibit fungal growth in storage environments.
	Cleaning and sorting	Removing contaminated grains or other materials through mechanical cleaning or manual sorting.
Biological control	Competitive exclusion	Using beneficial fungi or bacteria to outcompete mycotoxin-producing fungi in the field or storage.
	Biocontrol agents	Applying non-toxic microorganisms (e.g., yeasts, bacteria) to inhibit the growth of mycotoxigenic fungi.
Detoxification	Chemical decontamination	Applying chemicals like ammonia or ozone to degrade mycotoxins in contaminated crops.
	Biological detoxification	Using enzymes or microbes capable of breaking down or binding mycotoxins into less harmful forms.
	Adsorbents	Adding materials (e.g., clay, activated charcoal) to animal feed to bind mycotoxins and prevent their absorption.
Processing interventions	Heat treatment	Using thermal processing (e.g., roasting, extrusion) to reduce mycotoxin levels in food and feed.
	Milling and dehulling	Removing outer layers of grains (where mycotoxins may concentrate) to reduce contamination levels.
	Fermentation	Employing fermentation processes (e.g., lactic acid bacteria) to degrade or bind mycotoxins in food.
Regulatory and monitoring	Testing and screening	Regular testing of crops, feed, and food products for mycotoxin levels to ensure safety compliance.
	Legal limits and standards	Government regulations enforcing maximum permissible levels of mycotoxins in food and feed products.
	Traceability and certification	Ensuring supply chain transparency and certifying products as mycotoxin-free through reliable sources.

Table 1.
Mycotoxin control strategies.

timely harvesting, and regular monitoring of crops for signs of fungal infection [84]. Educating farmers about GAP and providing resources and training are crucial steps in minimizing pre-harvest mycotoxin risks [85].

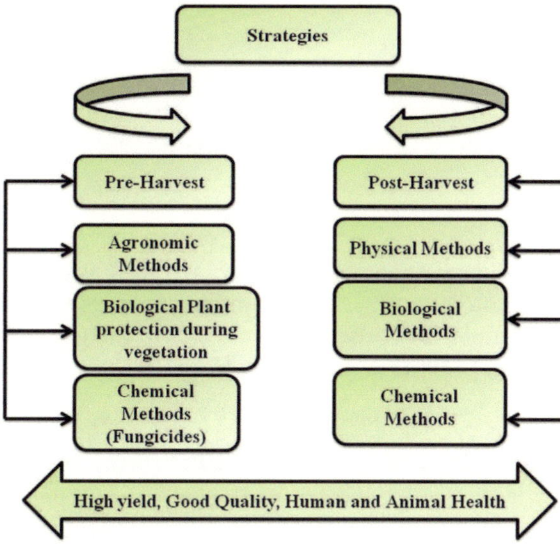

Figure 3.
Strategies of mycotoxins mitigation.

5.3 Post-harvest interventions

These interventions, critical for preventing mycotoxin contamination during storage and processing, include:

- *Proper drying*: Ensuring crops are adequately dried before storage to prevent fungal growth [86].
- *Controlled storage conditions:* Maintaining optimal storage conditions, such as low humidity and temperature, to prevent fungal growth [87].
- *Sorting and cleaning:* Removing damaged or moldy grains through sorting and cleaning processes to reduce mycotoxin levels [88].
- *Use of antifungal agents:* Applying antifungal agents to inhibit fungal growth during storage [89].

5.4 Biological control

This strategy uses living organisms, such as non-toxigenic fungi, bacteria, or yeast, to reduce mycotoxin-producing fungi [90]. For example, the use of non-toxigenic strains that compete with toxigenic strains can reduce aflatoxin contamination in crops like maize and peanuts [91].

5.5 Chemical and physical detoxification

Detoxification methods can be employed to decrease mycotoxin levels in food and feed [92]. These include chemical detoxification using agents like ammonia or sodium bisulfite, and physical methods such as heat treatment or irradiation [93].

5.6 Genetic engineering

Advances in genetic engineering offer promising avenues for reducing mycotoxin contamination [94]. This involves introducing genes that confer resistance to fungal colonization or mycotoxin biosynthesis into crop plants [95].

5.7 Mycotoxin binders

In the animal feed industry, mycotoxin binders are used as feed additives to reduce the bioavailability of mycotoxins [96]. These binders, composed of clay minerals, yeast cell walls, or other materials, adsorb mycotoxins in the gastrointestinal tract of animals, preventing their absorption and toxic effects [97].

6. Regulatory frameworks and international standards

The global nature of food trade requires a coordinated approach to mycotoxin regulation [98]. Different countries and international organizations have established regulatory frameworks and standards to protect consumers from mycotoxin exposure [99].

6.1 Codex alimentarius

The Codex Alimentarius, established jointly by the Food and Agriculture Organization (FAO) and the World Health Organization (WHO), sets international food standards, including those for mycotoxins [100]. Codex standards serve as the main principles for countries in establishing their own regulations and for resolving trade disputes related to food safety [101]. The Codex Alimentarius has set up the maximum permissible levels for several mycotoxins in various food products, including aflatoxins in peanuts and maize, and ochratoxin A in cereals and coffee [13, 102].

6.2 National regulations

Many countries have developed their own regulations and monitoring systems to control mycotoxin levels in food and feed [103]. These regulations often specify maximum allowable levels of mycotoxins in different commodities, based on risk assessments conducted by national food safety authorities [104]. For example:

- *United States:* The U.S. Food and Drug Administration (FDA) has established regulatory limits for aflatoxins in various food products, permitting only up to 20 parts per billion (ppb) in foods for human consumption [105].

- *European Union:* The European Union (EU) has implemented stringent regulations on mycotoxins, setting the maximum tolerable levels for various mycotoxins in food and feed set by the European Commission. The EU's Rapid Alert System for Food and Feed (RASFF) is also used to monitor and respond to mycotoxin contamination incidents [106].

- *China:* China has established maximum levels for several mycotoxins, including aflatoxins and ochratoxins, in food products [107]. The country's regulatory framework aims to protect public health and ensure the safety of exported food products.

6.3 Challenges in harmonization

Despite the existence of international standards, there are significant challenges in harmonizing mycotoxin regulations across different countries [22, 98]. Variations in climate, agricultural practices, and dietary habits can influence the levels of mycotoxins in food and the associated health risks [108]. As a result, countries may adopt different regulatory thresholds, which can create barriers to international trade.

6.4 Role of monitoring and surveillance programs

Effective monitoring and surveillance programs are essential for ensuring compliance with mycotoxin regulations and protecting public health [8, 23]. These programs involve the routine testing of food and feed samples for mycotoxin contamination, as well as the investigation of outbreaks of mycotoxin-related illnesses [109]. Advanced analytical methods, such as HPLC-MS, play a critical role in these programs by providing accurate and reliable data on mycotoxin levels [110].

6.5 Consumer awareness and education

Raising consumer awareness about mycotoxins and their potential health risks is an important component of food safety efforts [70]. Public education campaigns increase food literacy and help the public to make informed choices about the foods they purchase and consume, as well as encourage them to adopt practices that reduce the risk of mycotoxin exposure, such as proper food storage and preparation [111].

7. Future directions in mycotoxin research and control

The field of mycotoxin research is dynamic, with ongoing efforts to better understand the mechanisms of mycotoxin production, improve detection methods, and develop more effective strategies for mycotoxin control [112].

7.1 Omics technologies

The application of omics technologies, such as genomics, proteomics, and metabolomics, is providing new insights into the biology of mycotoxin-producing fungi [113, 114]. These technologies are helping researchers identify the genes and metabolic pathways involved in mycotoxin biosynthesis, as well as the environmental and biological factors that regulate their expression [115]. Such knowledge could lead to the development of targeted interventions that disrupt mycotoxin production at the molecular level [68].

7.2 Climate change and mycotoxin risk

Climate change has purportedly impacted the prevalence and distribution of mycotoxins [116]. Temperature fluctuations, changed precipitation patterns, and extreme weather events can alter the growth and toxin production of fungi, potentially leading to increased mycotoxin contamination in certain regions [27]. Understanding the interactions between climate change and mycotoxin risk is a growing area of research that will be critical for developing adaptive strategies to ensure food safety in a changing climate [117].

7.3 Sustainable agriculture

Sustainable agricultural practices are increasingly being recognized as a key component of mycotoxin control. Integrated pest management (IPM), crop diversification, and the use of organic farming methods can reduce the risk of fungal contamination and mycotoxin production [118]. Research into the development of sustainable farming practices that are both effective and economically viable will be important for reducing the global burden of mycotoxins [119].

7.4 Global collaboration and capacity building

Addressing the global challenge of mycotoxins requires collaboration across borders and disciplines [120]. International partnerships, such as those facilitated by the FAO, WHO, and other organizations, are essential for sharing knowledge, resources, and best practices [121]. Capacity-building initiatives, particularly in developing countries, are also crucial for improving mycotoxin management and ensuring food safety worldwide [122].

7.5 Innovative approaches to detoxification

Research into new methods of mycotoxin detoxification continues to advance, with promising approaches emerging in areas such as enzymatic degradation, microbial detoxification, and the use of nanoparticles [123]. These innovative technologies have the potential to complement existing detoxification strategies and provide more effective solutions for mitigating mycotoxin poisoning in food and feed [124].

8. Conclusion

The issue of mycotoxin contamination is a complex and serious challenge that requires a coordinated and multidisciplinary approach [16]. Progress has been made in understanding the environmental and biological factors that drive mycotoxin production, developing advanced detection methods, and implementing effective mitigation strategies to safeguard food safety [125]. However, new challenges, particularly due to climate change and global trade, require ongoing research and innovation to stay ahead of the risks posed by mycotoxins [126]. The future of mycotoxin research and control depends on integrating advanced technologies, sustainable agricultural practices, and global collaboration [16]. By pushing the boundaries of scientific knowledge and leveraging international cooperation, we can work toward minimizing the threat of mycotoxin contamination and ensuring safe and nutritious food for all [127].

DOI: http://dx.doi.org/10.5772/intechopen.1008400

Author details

Preeti Kaur[1] and Shubhankar Anand[2*]

1 Design Innovation Center, University of Delhi, New Delhi, India

2 School of Biomedical Sciences, Galgotias University, Greater Noida, Uttar Pradesh, India

*Address all correspondence to: shubhankar.anand@galgotiasuniversity.edu.in

References

[1] Köhler JR et al. Fungi that infect humans. Microbiology Spectrum. 2017;**5**(3). DOI: 10.1128/microbiolspec.funk-0014-2016

[2] Tedersoo L et al. Global diversity and geography of soil fungi. Science. 2014;**346**(6213):1256688

[3] Zain ME. Impact of mycotoxins on humans and animals. Journal of Saudi Chemical Society. 2011;**15**(2):129-144

[4] Omotayo OP et al. Prevalence of mycotoxins and their consequences on human health. Toxicological Research. 2019;**35**:1-7

[5] Newell DG et al. Food-borne diseases—The challenges of 20 years ago still persist while new ones continue to emerge. International Journal of Food Microbiology. 2010;**139**:S3-S15

[6] El-Sayed RA et al. An overview on the major mycotoxins in food products: Characteristics, toxicity, and analysis. Journal of Future Foods. 2022;**2**(2):91-102

[7] Dragan M et al. Climate change: Impact on mycotoxins incidence and food safety. Теория и практика переработки мяса. 2019;**4**(1):9-16

[8] Chilaka CA et al. Mycotoxin regulatory status in Africa: A decade of weak institutional efforts. Toxins. 2022;**14**(7):442

[9] Imran M et al. Mycotoxins–a global one health concern: A review. Agrobiological Records. 2020;**2**:1-16

[10] Richard JL. Some major mycotoxins and their mycotoxicoses—An overview. International Journal of Food Microbiology. 2007;**119**(1-2):3-10

[11] Asim M et al. Role of aflatoxin B1 as a risk for primary liver cancer in north Indian population. Clinical Biochemistry. 2011;**44**(14-15):1235-1240

[12] Waśkiewicz A, Beszterda M, Goliński P. Occurrence of fumonisins in food–an interdisciplinary approach to the problem. Food Control. 2012;**26**(2):491-499

[13] Eskola M et al. Worldwide contamination of food-crops with mycotoxins: Validity of the widely cited 'FAO estimate'of 25%. Critical Reviews in Food Science and Nutrition. 2020;**60**(16):2773-2789

[14] Agriopoulou S, Stamatelopoulou E, Varzakas T. Advances in occurrence, importance, and mycotoxin control strategies: Prevention and detoxification in foods. Food. 2020;**9**(2):137

[15] Zingales V et al. Climate change and effects on molds and mycotoxins. Toxins. 2022;**14**(7):445

[16] Fumagalli F et al. Integrated mycotoxin management system in the feed supply chain: Innovative approaches. Toxins. 2021;**13**(8):572

[17] Wu F. Mycotoxin risks are lower in biotech corn. Current Opinion in Biotechnology. 2022;**78**:102792

[18] Singh J, Mehta A. Rapid and sensitive detection of mycotoxins by advanced and emerging analytical methods: A review. Food Science and Nutrition. 2020;**8**(5):2183-2204

[19] Agriopoulou S, Stamatelopoulou E, Varzakas T. Advances in analysis and detection of major mycotoxins in foods. Food. 2020;**9**(4):518

[20] Wang Y et al. Recent progress in rapid determination of mycotoxins based on emerging biorecognition molecules: A review. Toxins. 2022;**14**(2):73

[21] Zadravec M et al. Biocontrol methods in avoidance and downsizing of mycotoxin contamination of food crops. PRO. 2022;**10**(4):655

[22] Dohlman E. Mycotoxin hazards and regulations. International Trade and Food Safety. 2003;**97**

[23] López-García R. Mycotoxin management: An international challenge. In: Ensuring Global Food Safety. Elsevier; 2022. pp. 213-219

[24] Rauwane ME et al. Pathogenicity and virulence factors of *Fusarium graminearum* including factors discovered using next generation sequencing technologies and proteomics. Microorganisms. 2020;**8**(2):305

[25] Paterson RRM, Lima N. Further mycotoxin effects from climate change. Food Research International. 2011;**44**(9):2555-2566

[26] Chhaya RS, O'Brien J, Cummins E. Feed to fork risk assessment of mycotoxins under climate change influences-recent developments. Trends in Food Science and Technology. 2022;**126**:126-141

[27] Casu A et al. Changing climate, shifting mycotoxins: A comprehensive review of climate change impact on mycotoxin contamination. Comprehensive Reviews in Food Science and Food Safety. 2024;**23**(2):e13323

[28] Wijerathna-Yapa A, Pathirana R. Sustainable agro-food systems for addressing climate change and food security. Agriculture. 2022;**12**(10):1554

[29] Adeyeye SO, Ashaolu T, Idowu-Adebayo F. Mycotoxins: Food safety, consumer health and Africa's food security. Polycyclic Aromatic Compounds. 2022;**42**(8):5779-5795

[30] Leach WD, Pelkey NW, Sabatier PA. Stakeholder partnerships as collaborative policymaking: Evaluation criteria applied to watershed management in California and Washington. Journal of Policy Analysis and Management: The Journal of the Association for Public Policy Analysis and Management. 2002;**21**(4):645-670

[31] Puri S, Shingh S, Tiwari P. Mycotoxins: A threat to food security and health. International Journal of Applied Sciences and Biotechnology. 2019;**7**(3):298-303

[32] Nielsen KF et al. Review of secondary metabolites and mycotoxins from the aspergillus Niger group. Analytical and Bioanalytical Chemistry. 2009;**395**:1225-1242

[33] Nesic K, Ivanovic S, Nesic V. Fusarial toxins: Secondary metabolites of *Fusarium fungi*. Reviews of Environmental Contamination and Toxicology. 2013;**228**:101-120

[34] Cano P, Puel O, Oswald IP. Mycotoxins: Fungal secondary metabolites with toxic properties. In: Fungi. CRC Press; 2018. pp. 318-371

[35] Ramadan NA, Al-Ameri HA. Aflatoxins, in Aflatoxins-Occurrence, Detoxification, Determination and Health Risks. London, UK: IntechOpen; 2022

[36] Petzinger E, Weidenbach A. Mycotoxins in the food chain: The role of ochratoxins. Livestock Production Science. 2002;**76**(3):245-250

[37] Scott P. Recent research on fumonisins: A review. Food Additives and Contaminants: Part A. 2012;**29**(2):242-248

[38] Tola M, Kebede B. Occurrence, importance and control of mycotoxins: A review. Cogent Food and Agriculture. 2016;**2**(1):1191103

[39] Schatzmayr G, Streit E. Global occurrence of mycotoxins in the food and feed chain: Facts and figures. World Mycotoxin Journal. 2013;**6**(3):213-222

[40] Klich MA. *Aspergillus flavus*: The major producer of aflatoxin. Molecular Plant Pathology. 2007;**8**(6):713-722

[41] Gourama H, Bullerman LB. *Aspergillus flavus* and aspergillus parasiticus: Aflatoxigenic fungi of concern in foods and feeds: A review. Journal of Food Protection. 1995;**58**(12):1395-1404

[42] Rushing BR, Selim MI. Aflatoxin B1: A review on metabolism, toxicity, occurrence in food, occupational exposure, and detoxification methods. Food and Chemical Toxicology. 2019;**124**:81-100

[43] Ogodo AC, Ugbogu OC. Public health significance of aflatoxin in food industry—A review. European Journal of Clinical and Biomedical Sciences. 2016;**2**(5):51-58

[44] Bayman P et al. Ochratoxin production by the aspergillus ochraceus group and *Aspergillus alliaceus*. Applied and Environmental Microbiology. 2002;**68**(5):2326-2329

[45] Pitt JI. *Penicillium viridicatum*, *Penicillium verrucosum*, and production of ochratoxin A. Applied and Environmental Microbiology. 1987;**53**(2):266-269

[46] Cabañes FJ, Bragulat MR, Castellá G. Ochratoxin a producing species in the genus *Penicillium*. Toxins. 2010;**2**(5):1111-1120

[47] Joshi V, Pandit A, Vaidya D. Ochratoxin a in food: An overview. International Journal of Food and Fermentation Technology. 2017;**7**(1):13-24

[48] Malir F et al. Ochratoxin A: 50 years of research. Toxins. 2016;**8**(7):191

[49] Apaliya MT et al. The occurrence of Ochratoxin A in food and its risk to human. In: Microbial Toxins in Food Systems: Causes, Mechanisms, Complications, and Metabolism. Springer; 2024. pp. 361-372

[50] Fandohan P et al. Infection of maize by Fusarium species and contamination with fumonisin in Africa. African Journal of Biotechnology. 2003;**2**(12):570-579

[51] Smith GW. Fumonisins. In: Veterinary Toxicology. Elsevier; 2018. pp. 1003-1018

[52] Hueza IM et al. Zearalenone, an estrogenic mycotoxin, is an immunotoxic compound. Toxins. 2014;**6**(3):1080-1095

[53] Luo S et al. Contamination status of major mycotoxins in agricultural product and food stuff in Europe. Food Control. 2021;**127**:108120

[54] Balló A et al. Estrogenic and non-estrogenic disruptor effect of zearalenone on male reproduction: A review. International Journal of Molecular Sciences. 2023;**24**(2):1578

[55] Placinta C, D'Mello JF, Macdonald A. A review of worldwide contamination of cereal grains and animal feed with Fusarium mycotoxins. Animal

Feed Science and Technology. 1999;**78**(1-2):21-37

[56] Sobrova P et al. Deoxynivalenol and its toxicity. Interdisciplinary Toxicology. 2010;**3**(3):94-99

[57] Aguzey HA et al. The effects of deoxynivalenol (DON) on the gut microbiota, morphology and immune system of chicken–a review. Annals of Animal Science. 2019;**19**(2):305-318

[58] Mannaa M, Kim KD. Influence of temperature and water activity on deleterious fungi and mycotoxin production during grain storage. Mycobiology. 2017;**45**(4):240-254

[59] Milani J. Ecological conditions affecting mycotoxin production in cereals: A review. Veterinární Medicína. 2013;**58**(8)

[60] Edwards SG. Influence of agricultural practices on Fusarium infection of cereals and subsequent contamination of grain by trichothecene mycotoxins. Toxicology Letters. 2004;**153**(1):29-35

[61] Nadeem F, Nawaz A, Farooq M. Crop Rotations, Fallowing, and Associated Environmental Benefits, in Oxford Research Encyclopedia of Environmental Science. 2019.

[62] Jacobsen BJ. Good agricultural and harvest practices to reduce mycotoxin contamination in wheat in temperate countries. Mycotoxin Reduction in Grain Chains. 2014:209-219

[63] Bilgrami KS, Choudhary AK. Mycotoxins in preharvest contamination of agricultural crops. In: Mycotoxins in Agriculture and Food Safety. CRC Press; 1998. pp. 19-62

[64] Neme K, Mohammed A. Mycotoxin occurrence in grains and the role of postharvest management as a mitigation strategies. A Review. Food Control. 2017;**78**:412-425

[65] Kaaya AN, Kyamuhangire W. The effect of storage time and agroecological zone on mould incidence and aflatoxin contamination of maize from traders in Uganda. International Journal of Food Microbiology. 2006;**110**(3):217-223

[66] Negash D. A review of aflatoxin: Occurrence, prevention, and gaps in both food and feed safety. Journal of Applied Microbiological Research;**1**(1):35-43

[67] Gbashi S et al. The socio-economic impact of mycotoxin contamination in Africa. Mycotoxins-Impact and Management Strategies. 2018

[68] Alberts J et al. Technological and community-based methods to reduce mycotoxin exposure. Food Control. 2017;**73**:101-109

[69] Tesfamariam K et al. Dietary mycotoxins exposure and child growth, immune system, morbidity, and mortality: A systematic literature review. Critical Reviews in Food Science and Nutrition. 2020;**60**(19):3321-3341

[70] Wagacha J, Muthomi J. Mycotoxin problem in Africa: Current status, implications to food safety and health and possible management strategies. International Journal of Food Microbiology. 2008;**124**(1):1-12

[71] Turner NW, Subrahmanyam S, Piletsky SA. Analytical methods for determination of mycotoxins: A review. Analytica Chimica Acta. 2009;**632**(2):168-180

[72] Kong W-J et al. Development of a sensitive and reliable high performance liquid chromatography method with fluorescence detection for

high-throughput analysis of multi-class mycotoxins in Coix seed. Analytica Chimica Acta. 2013;**799**:68-76

[73] Medina DAV et al. Current role of modern chromatography and mass spectrometry in the analysis of mycotoxins in food. TrAC Trends in Analytical Chemistry. 2021;**135**:116156

[74] Nováková L, Svoboda P, Pavlík J. Ultra-high performance liquid chromatography. In: Liquid Chromatography. Elsevier; 2017. pp. 719-769

[75] Majdinasab M, Ben Aissa S, Marty JL. Advances in colorimetric strategies for mycotoxins detection: Toward rapid industrial monitoring. Toxins. 2020;**13**(1):13

[76] Tsolakis NK et al. Agrifood supply chain management: A comprehensive hierarchical decision-making framework and a critical taxonomy. Biosystems Engineering. 2014;**120**:47-64

[77] Peltomaa R, Benito-Peña E, Moreno-Bondi MC. Bioinspired recognition elements for mycotoxin sensors. Analytical and Bioanalytical Chemistry. 2018;**410**:747-771

[78] Vidal JC et al. Electrochemical affinity biosensors for detection of mycotoxins: A review. Biosensors and Bioelectronics. 2013;**49**:146-158

[79] Edwards SG, O'callaghan J, Dobson AD. PCR-based detection and quantification of mycotoxigenic fungi. Mycological Research. 2002;**106**(9):1005-1025

[80] Kanja C et al. Cereal-Fusarium Interactions: Improved Fundamental Insights into Fusarium Pathogenomics and Cereal Host Resistance Reveals New Ways to Achieve Durable Disease Control, in Achieving Durable Disease Resistance in Cereals. Burleigh Dodds Science Publishing; 2021. pp. 111-189

[81] Nada S et al. Prevention and practical strategies to control mycotoxins in the wheat and maize chain. Food Control. 2022;**136**:108855

[82] Bhatnagar-Mathur P et al. Biotechnological advances for combating *Aspergillus flavus* and aflatoxin contamination in crops. Plant Science. 2015;**234**:119-132

[83] Moretti A, Logrieco AF, Susca A. Mycotoxins: An underhand food problem. In: Mycotoxigenic Fungi: Methods and Protocols. 2017. pp. 3-12

[84] Bruns HA. Controlling aflatoxin and fumonisin in maize by crop management. Journal of Toxicology: Toxin Reviews. 2003;**22**(2-3):153-173

[85] Gachara G et al. Drivers of post-harvest aflatoxin contamination: Evidence gathered from knowledge disparities and field surveys of maize farmers in the rift valley region of Kenya. Toxins. 2022;**14**(9):618

[86] Bradford KJ et al. The dry chain: Reducing postharvest losses and improving food safety in humid climates. In: Food Industry Wastes. Elsevier; 2020. pp. 375-389

[87] Northolt MD, Bullerman LB. Prevention of mold growth and toxin production through control of environmental conditions. Journal of Food Protection. 1982;**45**(6):519-526

[88] Shi H, Stroshine RL, Ileleji K. Aflatoxin Reduction in Corn by Cleaning and Sorting. Montreal, Quebec Canada: American Society of Agricultural and Biological Engineers; 2014

[89] Leyva Salas M et al. Antifungal microbial agents for food biopreservation—A review. Microorganisms. 2017;**5**(3):37

[90] Sarrocco S, Vannacci G. Preharvest application of beneficial fungi as a strategy to prevent postharvest mycotoxin contamination: A review. Crop Protection. 2018;**110**:160-170

[91] Ehrlich KC. Non-aflatoxigenic *Aspergillus flavus* to prevent aflatoxin contamination in crops: Advantages and limitations. Frontiers in Microbiology. 2014;**5**:50

[92] Jard G et al. Review of mycotoxin reduction in food and feed: From prevention in the field to detoxification by adsorption or transformation. Food Additives and Contaminants: Part A. 2011;**28**(11):1590-1609

[93] Samarajeewa U et al. Detoxification of aflatoxins in foods and feeds by physical and chemical methods. Journal of Food Protection. 1990;**53**(6):489-501

[94] Rajasekaran K, Cary J, Cleveland T. Prevention of preharvest aflatoxin contamination through genetic engineering of crops. Mycotoxin Research. 2006;**22**:118-124

[95] Perincherry L, Lalak-Kańczugowska J, Stępień Ł. Fusarium-produced mycotoxins in plant-pathogen interactions. Toxins. 2019;**11**(11):664

[96] Kolosova A, Stroka J. Evaluation of the effect of mycotoxin binders in animal feed on the analytical performance of standardised methods for the determination of mycotoxins in feed. Food Additives and Contaminants: Part A. 2012;**29**(12):1959-1971

[97] Nadziakiewicza M, Kehoe S, Micek P. Physico-chemical properties of clay minerals and their use as a health promoting feed additive. Animals. 2019;**9**(10):714

[98] Van Egmond HP, Schothorst RC, Jonker MA. Regulations relating to mycotoxins in food: Perspectives in a global and European context. Analytical and Bioanalytical Chemistry. 2007;**389**:147-157

[99] Duarte S, Lino C, Pena A. Mycotoxin food and feed regulation and the specific case of ochratoxin A: A review of the worldwide status. Food Additives and Contaminants. 2010;**27**(10):1440-1450

[100] Van Egmond HP. Worldwide regulations for mycotoxins. In: Mycotoxins and Food Safety. Springer; 2002. pp. 257-269

[101] Roberts D, Unnevehr L. Resolving trade disputes arising from trends in food safety regulation: The role of the multilateral governance framework. World Trade Review. 2005;**4**(3):469-497

[102] Marrez DA, Ayesh AM. Mycotoxins: The threat to food safety. Egyptian Journal of Chemistry. 2022;**65**(1):353-372

[103] Kebede H et al. Current status of major mycotoxins contamination in food and feed in Africa. Food Control. 2020;**110**:106975

[104] Anukul N, Vangnai K, Mahakarnchanakul W. Significance of regulation limits in mycotoxin contamination in Asia and risk management programs at the national level. Journal of Food and Drug Analysis. 2013;**21**(3):227-241

[105] Robens J, Cardwell K. The costs of mycotoxin management to the USA: Management of aflatoxins in the United States. Journal of Toxicology: Toxin Reviews. 2003;**22**(2-3):139-152

[106] Alshannaq A, Yu J-H. Analysis of EU rapid alert system (RASFF) notifications for aflatoxins in exported US food and feed products for 2010-2019. Toxins. 2021;**13**(2):90

[107] Selvaraj JN et al. Recent mycotoxin survey data and advanced mycotoxin detection techniques reported from China: A review. Food Additives and Contaminants: Part A. 2015;**32**(4):440-452

[108] Medina A et al. Climate change, food security and mycotoxins: Do we know enough? Fungal Biology Reviews. 2017;**31**(3):143-154

[109] Imade F et al. Updates on food and feed mycotoxin contamination and safety in Africa with special reference to Nigeria. Mycology. 2021;**12**(4):245-260

[110] Capriotti AL et al. Multiclass mycotoxin analysis in food, environmental and biological matrices with chromatography/mass spectrometry. Mass Spectrometry Reviews. 2012;**31**(4):466-503

[111] Guthrie J, Mancino L, Lin CTJ. Nudging consumers toward better food choices: Policy approaches to changing food consumption behaviors. Psychology and Marketing. 2015;**32**(5):501-511

[112] Ngolong Ngea GL et al. Recent trends in detecting, controlling, and detoxifying of patulin mycotoxin using biotechnology methods. Comprehensive Reviews in Food Science and Food Safety. 2020;**19**(5):2447-2472

[113] Eshelli M et al. Current status and future opportunities of omics tools in mycotoxin research. Toxins. 2018;**10**(11):433

[114] Wijayawardene NN et al. OMICS and other advanced technologies in mycological applications. Journal of Fungi. 2023;**9**(6):688

[115] Kolawole O et al. A review of mycotoxin biosynthetic pathways: Associated genes and their expressions under the influence of climatic factors. Fungal Biology Reviews. 2021;**37**:8-26

[116] Berry JP. Toxicology and climate change. In: Toxicology for the Health and Pharmaceutical Sciences. CRC Press; 2021. pp. 411-448

[117] Tirado MC et al. Climate change and food safety: A review. Food Research International. 2010;**43**(7):1745-1765

[118] Vasileiadis V et al. Crop protection in European maize-based cropping systems: Current practices and recommendations for innovative integrated pest management. Agricultural Systems. 2011;**104**(7):533-540

[119] Drakopoulos D et al. The agronomic and economic viability of innovative cropping systems to reduce Fusarium head blight and related mycotoxins in wheat. Agricultural Systems. 2021;**192**:103198

[120] Leslie J et al. The MyToolbox EU–China partnership—Progress and future directions in mycotoxin research and management. Toxins. 2020;**12**(11):712

[121] Eruaga MA. Enhancing Global Food Safety Standards through International Collaboration and Policy Harmonization. 2024.

[122] Ortega-Beltran A, Bandyopadhyay R. Contributions of integrated aflatoxin management strategies to achieve the sustainable development goals in various African countries. Global Food Security. 2021;**30**:100559

[123] Zhang X et al. Recent advances on emerging nanomaterials for controlling the mycotoxin contamination: From detection to elimination. Food Frontiers. 2020;**1**(4):360-381

[124] Zhu Y et al. Innovative technologies for the mitigation of mycotoxins in animal feed and ingredients—A review of recent patents. Animal Feed Science and Technology. 2016;**216**:19-29

[125] Li T et al. The occurrence and management of fumonisin contamination across the food production and supply chains. Journal of Advanced Research. 2024;**60**:13-26

[126] Montet D et al. Mycotoxins in Food and Beverages: Innovations and Advances Part I. CRC Press; 2021

[127] Chávez-Dulanto PN et al. Increasing the impact of science and technology to provide more people with healthier and safer food. Food and Energy Security. 2021;**10**(1):e259

Chapter 2

Detection and Detoxification Methods for Mycotoxins: From Classical to New Trends

Ahmet Düzel

Abstract

Mycotoxins are toxic secondary metabolites produced by certain filamentous fungi. Hundreds of mycotoxins have been identified to date, and these mycotoxins have adversely affected human and animal health, as well as agriculture and the economy. Indeed, mycotoxin contamination in food and feed is pervasive and causes significant losses every year. As complete prevention of mycotoxin formation is close to impossible, researchers are actively developing new detection and detoxification techniques. In addition, mycotoxin detection methods often require some pretreatments for accurate measurement. On the other hand, in addition to physical, chemical and biological methods, mycotoxins can also be detoxified by other methods that have emerged in recent years. This study aims to highlight the detection and detoxification methods for mycotoxins and introduce innovative approaches in these areas.

Keywords: mycotoxins, detection, detoxification, classical, new trends

1. Introduction

Mycotoxin is derived from the terms "myco" meaning "fungus" and "toxin" meaning poison. Mycotoxins are potentially hazardous secondary metabolites produced by some types of filamentous fungi (molds) genera such as Aspergillus, Penicillium, Fusarium, Alternaria and Claviceps. Mycotoxins are the most toxic chemical agents found in food and feed, posing the greatest threat to human and animal health [1, 2]. More than 300 mycotoxins have been identified to date, the most common of which are aflatoxins, ochratoxins, fumonisins, trichothecenes (T2, DON, DAS, HT2), ergot alkaloids, alternaria, patulin, citrinin and zearalenone toxins are the most important mycotoxins related to agriculture, economics, and public health [2].

Mycotoxin contamination is undesirable in all foods. However, attaining this goal through natural and artificial methods is not feasible, and a relatively small amount of these mycotoxins will always be present. Each year mycotoxin contamination of food and feedstuff causes heavy losses worldwide at the level of humans, animals, agriculture, and industries. So widespread is the contamination, researchers are making a strong effort to develop new techniques for the detection and detoxification of mycotoxins [3].

Detection of mycotoxins may require some pretreatments such as liquid-liquid and solid-liquid extraction, supercritical fluid extraction, filtration, gel chromatography and immune affinity purification. The analytical methods most commonly used to determine mycotoxin presence are high-performance liquid chromatography (HPLC), liquid chromatography combined with mass spectrometry (LC/MS), gas chromatography (GC), gas chromatography combined with mass spectrometry (GC/MS), Enzyme-Linked Immunosorbent Assay (ELISA) and quick tests [4].

Mycotoxin detoxification can be achieved by using physical methods, chemical methods, biological methods and other emerging methods. In addition, there are approaches to examine the effects of some of these emerging technologies on mycotoxin detoxification by combining them with fermentation [5]. This study, aims to introduce the detection and detoxification methods of mycotoxins and new approaches toward these methods.

2. Pretreatments for mycotoxin detection

Pretreatments allow mycotoxins in food samples with complex biochemical structures to be isolated by improving their concentration and purity. This minimizes the risk of instrument contamination, signal interference and matrix effects in the analytical detection methods to be applied in the next steps (**Figure 1**).

2.1 Extraction

Extraction of mycotoxins from food samples is the first step in sample preparation. For the isolation of mycotoxins, liquid foods such as fruit juice, wine and milk are subjected to liquid-liquid extraction (LLE), while solid foods such as cereals and grains are subjected to solid-liquid extraction (SLE). Most mycotoxins are highly soluble in organic solvents such as methanol, acetonitrile (ACN), acetone, dichloromethane and ethyl acetate, while (with the exception of fumonisins and patulin) they are only slightly soluble in water. To improve extraction efficiency, certain amounts of acidic buffer or water are often added to organic solvents. Recently, many instrumental solvent extraction methods such as supercritical fluid extraction (SFE), microwave-assisted extraction (MAE) and accelerated solvent extraction (ASE) have been used in mycotoxin analysis. Although these methods offer lower chemical solvent consumption and better extraction efficiency, these devices are costly and not easily available in common laboratories [6].

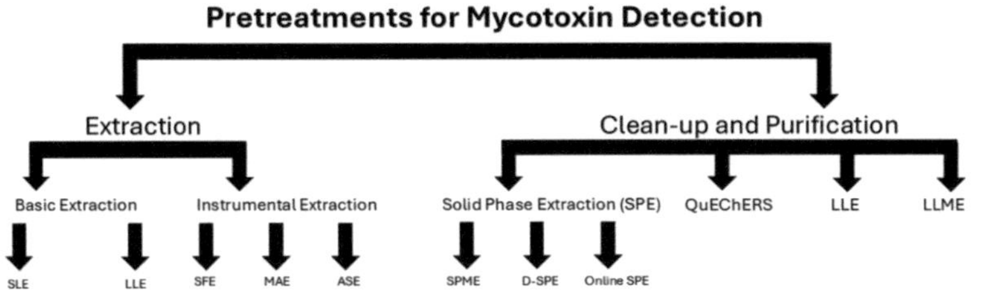

Figure 1.
Various pretreatments for the detection of mycotoxins.

2.2 Clean-up and purification

After extraction, filtration and centrifugation can be applied to remove coarse impurities before performing further clean-up steps. In the further clean-up steps, different techniques such as solid phase extraction (SPE), solid phase micro extraction (SPME), dispersive solid phase extraction (D-SPE), QuEChERS (quick, easy, cheap, effective, rugged and safe), liquid-liquid extraction (LLE), dispersive liquid-liquid micro extraction (DLLME) can be applied.

2.2.1 Solid-phase extraction (SPE)

SPE has been recognized as a beneficial alternative to classic liquid-liquid extraction due to the avoidance of large solvent consumption, tedious process and long operation time. With the development of SPE, new perspectives and progress are provided as methodological solutions in mycotoxin analysis. Significant progress has been observed in the simplification, automation and miniaturization of the original formats [7].

The adsorbent is the most important factor of the SPE method. According to the polarity of materials, commercial SPE adsorbents can be classified into four categories: (1) reversed-phase adsorbents for non-polar or weakly polar compounds, such as C18 and C8, (2) positive-phase adsorbents for polar compounds, such as CN, NH2 and Florisil, (3) ion-exchange adsorbents, such as SAX, PRS, and PSA, and (4) additional adsorbents, such as Oasis Hydrophilic Lipophilic Balance (HLB) and immunoaffinity columns (IACs). Apart from these, there are different adsorbents such as molecular recognition-based polymers (such as molecularly imprinted polymers and aptamers), nanoparticles-based adsorbents (such as graphene and its composites, activated carbon and its composites), bonded silica-based adsorbents (such as humic acid bound silica), hyper crosslinked polymers (such as synthesized from heterocyclic phenyl-imidazole monomers) which are being studied and promising [8].

2.2.1.1 Solid phase micro extraction (SPME) techniques

Since SPME combines sampling, extraction, sample cleaning and enrichment in a single step, it is one of the most simple and effective techniques. The efficiency of SPME has been supported further by the development of matrix-compatible coatings in which sorbent particles of a few or tens of μm in diameter are embedded in a polymeric binder like polyacrylonitrile (PAN). In these coatings, the binder forms a thin film that allows extraction and enrichment of only small molecules while avoiding interaction with large molecules (such as protein and cell matter) from the sample matrix [9].

2.2.1.2 Dispersive solid-phase extraction (D-SPE) techniques

Dispersive SPE (d-SPE) improves sensitivity and reduces sorption time by allowing sorbents to interact directly and quickly with targets. It avoids issues like high backpressure or clogging found in conventional SPE. d-SPE can be used alone or with other methods and is commonly applied in mycotoxin analysis through two approaches: dispersive micro-SPE (D-μ-SPE) and magnetic SPE (m-SPE). D-μ-SPE uses small amounts of micro- or nanomaterials, making the properties of sorbents critical for the accurate and efficient detection of mycotoxins. Nanomaterials in

D-μ-SPE offer rapid extraction and high efficiency, overcoming issues like back-pressure, and are more cost-effective and time-saving compared to traditional SPE cartridges. To improve the mass transfer kinetics, ultrasonication or vortex can be applied as an assistive technique for D-μ-SPE. M-SPE, which eliminates the need for centrifugation or filtration, is widely used in mycotoxin analysis. It incorporates magnetic properties with functional materials, and its application in this field is more extensively studied than D-μ-SPE, using magnetized carbon nanoparticles, functionalized magnetic nanoparticles, and magnetized nanoporous materials [7].

2.2.1.3 Online SPE

SPE techniques can be combined with the online system, which provides some advantages. Analysis time, sample loss and the amount of solvent required can be reduced, as well as sensitivity, accuracy, and precision can be increased by eliminating personal errors [10, 11]. Furthermore, the online system allows partial or total automation of analytical steps with some special facilities such as automatic sample loading, washing of interference, analyte elution, separation and detection by the analytical system [12, 13].

2.2.2 QuEChERS

The QuEChERS (quick, easy, cheap, effective, rugged and safe) method is one of the most widely used methods for the extraction of both solid and liquid food samples. This method is fast and requires less use of solvents, so it is both economical and environmentally friendly (since it produces less waste). This method involves two steps. In the first step, a separation based on inorganic and organic phases can be obtained by using salt solution and solvent. Moreover, solvents together with salts allow the separation of analytes with different polarity. The second step includes the clean-up stage, using various absorbents such as C18 (Octadecyl silica), PSA (N-Propylethane-1,2-diamine) and SPE cartridge. C18 is used to remove non-polar compounds, and PSA is used to remove sugars, lipids and organic acid. However, in some cases, it may be preferable not to have a clean-up step in this method [14].

2.2.3 Liquid-liquid extraction (LLE)

Liquid–liquid extraction (LLE) utilizes the differing solubility of a toxin in an aqueous phase versus an immiscible organic phase to isolate the compound into one solvent, while leaving the remaining matrix in the other [15]. For example, solvents like hexane and cyclohexane are employed to eliminate non-polar impurities, such as lipids and cholesterol. This method is effective for various toxins and is suitable for small-scale preparations. However, it can be time-consuming and depends on the specific matrix and compounds being analyzed. Another drawback is the potential loss of samples due to adsorption onto glassware [16].

2.2.4 Liquid phase microextraction (LPME)

Recently, liquid phase microextraction (LPME) methods have gained popularity and are increasingly being utilized. In these LPME techniques, analytes are extracted from an aqueous solution (donor phase) into a μL–level of a water-immiscible organic solvent (acceptor phase). Single-drop microextraction, hollow fiber-LPME, and dispersive liquid-liquid microextraction (DLLME) are three primary types of LPME techniques. Of these, DLLME has gained significant attention since it was developed in 2006. Its main advantages include simplicity, high extraction recovery (ER), enrichment factor (EF) and speed. However, DLLME has drawbacks, including the use of toxic solvents and a time-consuming centrifugation process. To address these issues, new methods like air-assisted liquid-liquid microextraction, ultrasound-assisted DLLME and effervescence-assisted DLLME (EA-DLLME) have been developed [17].

3. Mycotoxin detection methods

3.1 Analytical methods

Different kinds of analytical approaches such as thin layer chromatography (TLC), gas chromatography (GC), high-performance liquid chromatography (HPLC) and liquid chromatography coupled with mass spectrometry (LC-MS) have been used for mycotoxins detection in various samples.

TLC is a basic method, but it is generally considered to be less practical or to have insufficient sensitivity compared to LC methods. Nevertheless, a small number of researchers are investigating this method as it still has uses in certain situations [18].

Gas chromatographic methods based on Flame Ionization Detector (FID), Electron Capture Detector (ECD) and Mass Spectrometry (MS) detection are widely used methods for the quantitative simultaneous determination of mycotoxins. These methods require a preliminary clean-up of extracts and pre-column derivatization of the purified extract with specific reagents. Mass spectrometry (MS), or tandem mass spectrometry (MS/MS), offers an advantage in confirming the identity of chromatographic peaks [19].

HPLC is the most popular method for analyzing mycotoxins in food and feed. It is a quantitative technique ideal for the online clean-up of sample extracts and can be paired with various detectors, such as DAD, UV and FLD [20]. Fluorescence detectors are undoubtedly the most sensitive among the modern HPLC sensors [21]. Although HPLC-FLD offers sufficient sensitivity, the presence of various interferences in sample matrixes limits their direct application in food samples [22].

LC-MS technique coupling of LC and MS provides a great opportunity for the analysis of mycotoxins. HPLC with MS detection eliminates the need for sample derivatization for fluorescence activity enhancement. Furthermore, the use of LC and tandem mass spectrometry enables a very selective and sensitive detection. Liquid chromatography–tandem mass spectrometry (LC-MS/MS) is a useful technique for the identification and quantification of chemicals such as mycotoxins. Before the mass spectrometer, HPLC will separate the sample into chemical compounds. Then mass spectrometer will ionize molecules and sort, and identify them according to their mass-to-charge ratio (m/z) (**Figure 2**) [23].

3.2 Mycotoxin sensors

Biosensors are analytical devices that detect and measure target molecules using biological recognition elements and a signal transducer. Recently, there have been

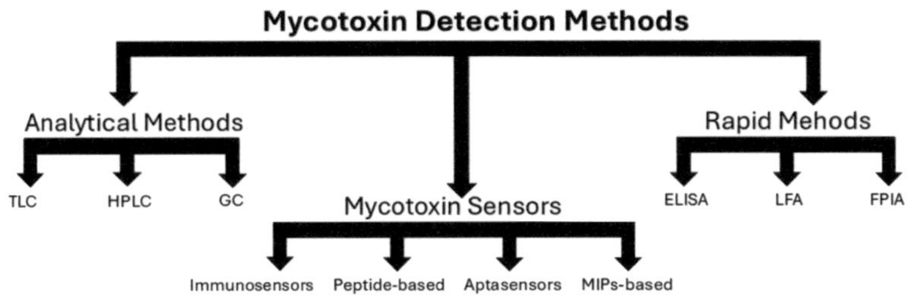

Figure 2.
Various methods for detection of mycotoxins.

efforts to develop different types of biosensors, including immunosensors, peptide-based sensors, aptasensors and molecularly imprinted polymer-based (MIPs-based) sensors for mycotoxin detection. They provide real-time monitoring of reactions by creating digital output formats. Mycotoxin screening methods can be advanced by improving sensitivity, robustness, simplicity and reusability. Various transducers for the development of mycotoxin sensors continue to be investigated, including electrochemical, calorimetric, optical and magnetic [24].

3.3 Rapid methods

3.3.1 Enzyme-linked immunosorbent assay (ELISA)

ELISA, developed by Engvall and Perlmann in 1971, is an immunological technique used to analyze protein samples in microplate wells with specific antibodies. The use of ELISA has become indispensable in food safety as well as in different fields over time. Typically conducted in 96-well plates, ELISA can involve direct labeling of targets or competitive binding with labeled secondary antibodies. Its simplicity, speed, high throughput, and low cost make it popular for rapid mycotoxin detection [25].

3.3.2 Lateral flow assay (LFA)

LFA-based instruments are ideal for rapid mycotoxin detection in food, providing results in 5–30 minutes without the need for complex preparation. These tools are stable, require minimal sample input and are user-friendly, making them accessible even in low-resource settings. Their portability and cost-effectiveness contribute to their growing popularity for on-site testing outside of laboratories. LFAs are categorized into sandwich and competitive types, with sandwich LFAs suited for larger molecules and competitive LFAs for smaller ones like mycotoxins [26].

3.3.3 Fluorescent polarization immunoassay (FPIA)

FPIA operates on the principle that exposing a fluorescent molecule in solution to polarized light at its excitation wavelength results in depolarized emission. Small fluorescent molecules rotate quickly and exhibit lower polarization, while their interaction with larger molecules like antibodies slows their rotation, increasing polarization. This increase can be measured, making it useful for developing competitive immunoassays for mycotoxin detection. In this competitive format, mycotoxins in the sample compete with a fluorophore-labeled tracer for binding sites on specific

Detection method	Advantages	Disadvantages
TLC	Quick, simple, and qualitative method	Low sensitivity and no quantification
HPLC	Good sensitivity, selectivity and repeatability, can be automated (autosampler), short analysis times, official methods available, provides confirmation (by different detectors).	Requirement expensive equipment, specialist expertise, pretreatment and derivatization.
GC	Simultaneous analysis, good sensitivity, can be automated (autosampler), provides confirmation (by different detectors).	Requirement expensive equipment, specialist expertise, pretreatment and derivatization. Matrix interference problems, calibration difficulties, variation in repeatability.
Sensors	Real time monitoring, suitable for development.	Cross-reactivity with related mycotoxins, (sometimes) clean-up needed, variation in repeatability.
ELISA	User-friendly, inexpensive equipment, high sensitivity, simultaneous analysis, suitable for screening, limited use of organic solvents.	Cross-reactivity with related mycotoxins, matrix interference problems, possible false results, confirmatory LC analysis required.
LFA	Rapid detection, no need complex preparation, require minimal sample input, user-friendly, no expensive equipment required.	Cross-reactivity with related mycotoxins, validation required for additional matrices.
FPIA	Rapid, no clean-up required.	Poor sensitivity in some cases, cross-reactivity with related mycotoxins, matrix interference problems.

Table 1.
Advantages and disadvantages of mycotoxin detection methods.

antibodies, affecting polarization levels. An increase in polarization indicates a negative sample, while a decrease signals the presence of mycotoxins, making polarization inversely proportional to their concentration (**Table 1**) [27].

4. Mycotoxin detoxification methods

4.1 Physical methods

Contaminated grain does not have the same color or density as safe grain. Thus, grain can be sorted according to appearance or density. In addition to basic sorting, the sieving cleaning technique can be applied by utilizing the size difference of the grains, and the flotation technique can be applied by utilizing the density difference. When mycotoxin contamination is heterogeneous, the removal of the contaminated portion may reduce the level of mycotoxin in the final product. Washing food or grain can also reduce mycotoxin levels. Indeed, water-soluble mycotoxins can be partially washed off the surface of grains. There are studies on the use of distilled water for this process, as well as the use of solutions with different contents [28].

The adsorption is another physical method applied for mycotoxin removal. The application of adsorption agents has become popular since the European Union (EU) allowed substrates that suppress or reduce the absorption, promote the excretion of mycotoxins or modify their mode of action to be used as feed additives [29].

Mycotoxins are generally very stable and are rarely eliminated by thermic treatment. Little or no reduction in mycotoxin levels occurs as a result of normal cooking conditions, such as boiling, frying. For efficiency of thermal processes, the initial level of contamination, type of mycotoxin and its concentration, heating temperature and time, the degree of heat penetration, moisture content, pH and ionic strength of the food all play a significant role in toxin degradation. Similarly, most mycotoxins are not often affected by irradiation. Radiolysis of water produces free radicals that could react with mycotoxins. In addition to UV, X and gamma-rays, microwave applications are also known to be effective in the detoxification of some mycotoxins [30].

Cold plasma is basically created by atmospheric dielectric discharge, with synthetic air as a working gas [31]. There are studies proving that cold plasma has antimicrobial and antimycotoxic effects on food surfaces. However, its potential cytotoxicity effect is still unclear because of the limited number of studies published [32].

4.2 Chemical methods

Various acidic, alkaline and oxidizing agent treatments have been used so far for the detoxification of mycotoxins. Some of these applications have also been supported by heating. Acids such as lactic acid, citric acid, hydrochloric acid have been used effectively in acidic treatments. For alkaline treatments, chemicals such as sodium hydroxide and ammonia have been used, with the most effective results obtained with ammonia. The use of ozone has also been widely involved in the detoxification of various mycotoxins. Although the results obtained in mycotoxin detoxification by chemical methods are highly successful, they have disadvantages such as the potential to form degradation products (conversion to another mycotoxin) and the high risk of producing chemical waste [33].

4.3 Biological methods

4.3.1 Microbial detoxifications

Microbial detoxification involves utilizing the metabolites or enzymes released by microorganisms during their growth, or the inherent traits of the microorganisms, to break down or inhibit the formation of mycotoxins, thus minimizing mycotoxin contamination. Additionally, microorganisms can directly adsorb mycotoxins from samples, aiding in their removal or reduction. Various wild-type bacterial species (especially lactic acid bacteria), yeasts (especially *Saccharomyces cerevisiae*), molds and actinomycetes can be employed for mycotoxin detoxification. With the rapid advancement of genetic engineering techniques, there are ongoing studies aimed at enhancing the detoxification abilities of these microorganisms [34–36].

4.3.2 Enzymatic detoxifications

Research into enzymes capable of converting mycotoxins into less harmful or non-toxic products has become increasingly significant. Various enzymes, such as laccase, manganese peroxidase (MnP) and oxidase, have been identified for this purpose. While identifying and purifying these mycotoxin-degrading enzymes (MDE) can be time-consuming and costly, using pure enzymes presents advantages over

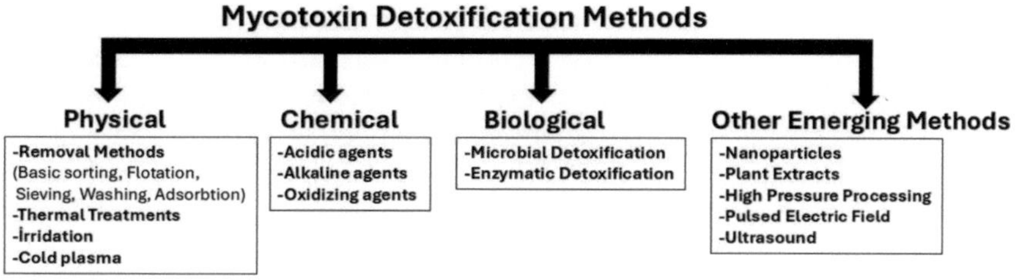

Figure 3.
Various methods for detoxification of mycotoxins.

whole bacterial cells, particularly in environments unsuitable for microbial survival. Enzymatic degradation offers benefits like ease of handling, consistent performance, high efficiency and specificity. However, many MDEs are stored intracellularly in fungi, making extraction challenging. Although some natural MDEs have been purified, their use in complex food and feed matrixes remains limited. Recombinant enzymes are particularly appealing because genetic engineering allows for efficient, cost-effective production. Recent studies have focused on enhancing yield and reducing purification costs, but commercial applications of recombinant MDEs are still not fully realized [37].

4.4 Other emerging methods

New approaches such as the use of nanoparticles and plant extracts are also being tested in mycotoxin detoxification. There are studies examining the effects of nanoparticles coated with some special substances (chitosan, etc.) to adsorb mycotoxins, inhibit mycotoxin-producing microorganisms and degrade mycotoxins. On the other hand, there are studies on the inactivation of mycotoxin-producing microorganisms and mycotoxins by components such as plant extracts, essential oils and secondary metabolites. Moreover, the use of plant extracts is attractive due to their extremely low toxicity and environmental friendliness compared to chemical methods [38].

High-pressure-processing (HPP), pulsed electric field (PEF), as well as ultrasound methods, have been identified as emerging and green technologies useful in controlling microorganisms and mycotoxins in foodstuffs. Using HPP, the structure of mycotoxins can be modified, which reduces both their toxicity and their ability to thrive in the environment. Moreover, this technique can be combined with moderate heating to deactivate heat-resistant microorganisms. PEF leads to a transmembrane voltage between the inner and outer parts of the cell membrane, which, after a certain point, leads to permanent structural changes and cell death. Although this method is more prominent in ensuring the death of mycotoxin-producing microorganisms in a short time, it has also been shown to be effective in mycotoxin degradation under some special conditions. The use of ultrasound has been shown to decontaminate cereal products and thereby prevent mycotoxin formation (**Figure 3**) [39].

5. Conclusion

Mycotoxins not only cause economic losses but also adversely affect human health. Moreover, the inevitability of mycotoxin formation in food products has necessitated the development of effective practices for the pre-production, during-production and post-production stages of food products. Therefore, rapid and accurate detection of mycotoxins and detoxification of mycotoxin-contaminated food products are of utmost importance. Although scientists have been working on both of these important factors for many years, due to the structural differences of each type of food product and mycotoxin, it has so far not been possible to determine the optimal type of detection and detoxification method, since it is not possible to obtain the same response after each treatment. Therefore, further studies on these issues and the development of new techniques remain important to shorten processing time, increase sensitivity and efficiency, and reduce processing costs. While it is encouraging that recent studies have shown promising results in these areas, the permanence of new techniques depends on meeting important criteria such as the absence of side effects and sustainable cost-effectiveness.

Author details

Ahmet Düzel
Environmental Engineering Department, Faculty of Engineering and Architecture, Sinop University, Sinop, Türkiye

*Address all correspondence to: ahmetduzel@gmail.com

References

[1] Atungulu G, Mohammadi-Shad Z. Reference on mycotoxins occurrence, prevalence, and risk assessment in food systems. In: Novel Technologies and Systems for Food Preservation. IGI Global; 2019. pp. 294-343

[2] El-Sayed RA, Jebur AB, Kang W, El-Demerdash FM. An overview on the major mycotoxins in food products: Characteristics, toxicity, and analysis. Journal of Future Foods. 2022;**2**(2):91-102

[3] Nahle S, El Khoury A, Assaf JC, Louka N, Chokr A, Atoui A. A promising innovative technique for mycotoxin detoxification from beverages using biofilms of lactic acid bacteria. Innovative Food Science and Emerging Technologies. 2022;**82**:103165

[4] Pleadin J, Frece J, Markov K. Mycotoxins in food and feed. Advances in Food and Nutrition Research. 2019;**89**:297-345

[5] Gavahian M, Mathad GN, Oliveira CA, Khaneghah AM. Combinations of emerging technologies with fermentation: Interaction effects for detoxification of mycotoxins. Food Research International. 2021;**141**:110104

[6] Yang Y, Li G, Wu D, Liu J, Li X, Luo P, et al. Recent advances on toxicity and determination methods of mycotoxins in foodstuffs. Trends in Food Science and Technology. 2020;**96**:233-252

[7] Tang Z, Liu F, Fang F, Ding X, Han Q, Tan Y, et al. Solid-phase extraction techniques based on nanomaterials for mycotoxin analysis: An overview for food and agricultural products. Journal of Separation Science. 2022;**45**(13):2273-2300

[8] Bian Y, Zhang Y, Zhou Y, Wei B, Feng X. Recent insights into sample pretreatment methods for mycotoxins in different food matrices: A critical review on novel materials. Toxins. 2023;**15**(3):215

[9] Zhou W, Wieczorek MN, Pawliszyn J. High throughput and automated solid-phase microextraction and determination by liquid chromatography-mass spectrometry for the analysis of mycotoxins in beer. Food Chemistry. 2023;**426**:136557

[10] Rodriguez-Mozaz S, de Alda MJL, Barceló D. Advantages and limitations of on-line solid phase extraction coupled to liquid chromatography–mass spectrometry technologies versus biosensors for monitoring of emerging contaminants in water. Journal of Chromatography A. 2007;**1152**(1-2):97-115

[11] Rogeberg M, Malerod H, Roberg-Larsen H, Aass C, Wilson SR. On-line solid phase extraction–liquid chromatography, with emphasis on modern bioanalysis and miniaturized systems. Journal of Pharmaceutical and Biomedical Analysis. 2014;**87**:120-129

[12] Campone L, Piccinelli AL, Celano R, Pagano I, Russo M, Rastrelli L. Rapid and automated on-line solid phase extraction HPLC–MS/MS with peak focusing for the determination of ochratoxin A in wine samples. Food Chemistry. 2018;**244**:128-135

[13] Maranata GJ, Surya NO, Hasanah AN. Optimising factors affecting solid phase extraction performances of molecular imprinted polymer as recent sample preparation technique. Heliyon. 2021;**7**(1)

[14] Sadighara P, Basaran B, Afshar A, Nazmara S. Optimization of clean-up in QuEChERS method for extraction of mycotoxins in food samples: A systematic review. Microchemical Journal. 2023;**109711**

[15] Razzazi-Fazeli E, Reiter EV. Sample preparation and clean up in mycotoxin analysis: Principles, applications and recent developments. Determining Mycotoxins and Mycotoxigenic Fungi in Food and Feed. 2011:37-70

[16] Turner NW, Subrahmanyam S, Piletsky SA. Analytical methods for determination of mycotoxins: A review. Analytica Chimica Acta. 2009;**632**(2):168-180

[17] Gholizadeh S, Mirzaei H, Khandaghi J, Mogaddam MRA, Javadi A. Ultrasound–assisted solvent extraction combined with magnetic ionic liquid based-dispersive liquid–liquid microextraction for the extraction of mycotoxins from tea samples. Journal of Food Composition and Analysis. 2022;**114**:104831

[18] Turner NW, Bramhmbhatt H, Szabo-Vezse M, Poma A, Coker R, Piletsky SA. Analytical methods for determination of mycotoxins: An update (2009-2014). Analytica Chimica Acta. 2015;**901**:12-33

[19] Pascale MN. Detection methods for mycotoxins in cereal grains and cereal products. Zbornik Matice srpske za prirodne nauke. 2009;**117**:15-25

[20] El-Zeiny SA, Taha MS, Abo El-Magd MK, Arafa MM, Badrawy NA, El-Rahman A, et al. Various analytical techniques involved in mycotoxin detection and estimation. Egyptian Journal of Chemistry and Environmental Health. 2015;**1**(1):729-748

[21] Singh J, Mehta A. Rapid and sensitive detection of mycotoxins by advanced and emerging analytical methods: A review. Food Science and Nutrition. 2020;**8**(5):2183-2204

[22] Rezaeefar A, Nemati M, Farajzadeh MA, Mogaddam MRA, Lotfipour F. Development of N and S doped carbon sorbent-based dispersive micro solid phase extraction method combined with dispersive liquid-liquid microextraction for selected mycotoxins from soymilk samples. Microchemical Journal. 2022;**173**:107039

[23] Rahmani A, Jinap S, Soleimany F. Qualitative and quantitative analysis of mycotoxins. Comprehensive Reviews in Food Science and Food Safety. 2009;**8**(3):202-251

[24] Khan R, Anwar F, Ghazali FM. A comprehensive review of mycotoxins: Toxicology, detection, and effective mitigation approaches. Heliyon. 2024

[25] Suo Z, Niu X, Wei M, Jin H, He B. Latest strategies for rapid and point of care detection of mycotoxins in food: A review. Analytica Chimica Acta. 2023;**1246**:340888

[26] Sadeghi P, Sohrabi H, Majidi MR, Eftekhari A, Zargari F, de la Guardia M, et al. Mycotoxins detection in food samples through lateral flow assays (LFAs)–an update for status and prospect. TrAC Trends in Analytical Chemistry. 2024;**117722**

[27] Nolan P, Auer S, Spehar A, Elliott CT, Campbell K. Current trends in rapid tests for mycotoxins. Food Additives and Contaminants: Part A. 2019;**36**(5):800-814

[28] Karlovsky P, Suman M, Berthiller F, De Meester J, Eisenbrand G, Perrin I, et al. Impact of food processing and

detoxification treatments on mycotoxin contamination. Mycotoxin Research. 2016;**32**:179-205

[29] Zhu Y, Hassan YI, Lepp D, Shao S, Zhou T. Strategies and methodologies for developing microbial detoxification systems to mitigate mycotoxins. Toxins. 2017;**9**(4):130

[30] Jard G, Liboz T, Mathieu F, Guyonvarc'h, A., and Lebrihi, A. Review of mycotoxin reduction in food and feed: From prevention in the field to detoxification by adsorption or transformation. Food Additives and Contaminants: Part A. 2011;**28**(11): 1590-1609

[31] Shanakhat H, Sorrentino A, Raiola A, Romano A, Masi P, Cavella S. Current methods for mycotoxins analysis and innovative strategies for their reduction in cereals: An overview. Journal of the Science of Food and Agriculture. 2018;**98**(11):4003-4013

[32] Gavahian M, Cullen PJ. Cold plasma as an emerging technique for mycotoxin-free food: Efficacy, mechanisms, and trends. Food Reviews International. 2020;**36**(2):193-214

[33] Aiko V, Mehta A. Occurrence, detection and detoxification of mycotoxins. Journal of Biosciences. 2015;**40**:943-954

[34] Abraham N, Chan ETS, Zhou T, Seah SY. Microbial detoxification of mycotoxins in food. Frontiers in Microbiology. 2022;**13**:957148

[35] McCormick SP. Microbial detoxification of mycotoxins. Journal of Chemical Ecology. 2013;**39**:907-918

[36] Xu H, Wang L, Sun J, Wang L, Guo H, Ye Y, et al. Microbial detoxification of mycotoxins in food and feed. Critical Reviews in Food Science and Nutrition. 2022;**62**(18):4951-4969

[37] Liu L, Xie M, Wei D. Biological detoxification of mycotoxins: Current status and future advances. International Journal of Molecular Sciences. 2022;**23**(3):1064

[38] Agriopoulou S, Stamatelopoulou E, Varzakas T. Advances in occurrence, importance, and mycotoxin control strategies: Prevention and detoxification in foods. Food. 2020;**9**(2):137

[39] Awuchi CG, Ondari EN, Ogbonna CU, Upadhyay AK, Baran K, Okpala COR, et al. Mycotoxins affecting animals, foods, humans, and plants: Types, occurrence, toxicities, action mechanisms, prevention, and detoxification strategies-A revisit. Food. 2021;**10**(6):1279

Chapter 3

Mycotoxins Diagnostic Methods from Past to Present

Leila Faeli

Abstract

Mycotoxins are toxic substances produced as byproducts of various types of mold. These mycotoxins are mainly linked to certain genera of fungi, such as *Aspergillus*, *Penicillium*, *Fusarium*, *Claviceps*, and *Alternaria*, and are formed under specific conditions. Mycotoxins encompass a range of chemically diverse compounds with a small molecular weight, typically less than 1000 Da. Currently, more than 500 mycotoxins are recognized as harmful to the health of humans, animals, and plants. Each type falls into particular groups with distinct toxic effects, with the most common and well-known ones being aflatoxins (AFTs), ochratoxins (OTs), fumonisins (FUMs), zearalenone (ZEN), trichothecenes (TCTs), patulin (PAT), and citrinin (CT). Adhering to good agricultural and industrial practices is crucial to reducing the risk of mycotoxin contamination in food production. Efficient and prompt detection of mycotoxins is of utmost importance in the realm of food safety. This chapter deals with conventional and commercial methods for mycotoxin detection from the past to the present.

Keywords: mycotoxins, fungal toxins, mycotoxicogenic, carcinogene, diagnostics

1. Introduction

Mycotoxins, which are toxic secondary metabolites, are produced by various types of fungi such as *Aspergillus*, *Penicillium*, *Fusarium*, and *Claviceps* and have the potential to infect crops before or after they are harvested. The growth of mold occurs under conditions that are dark and humid [1]. Mycotoxins can directly infect humans through contaminated food or indirectly through the contamination of livestock and their products. Foods such as grains, alcoholic beverages, nuts, sugar, cheeses, coffee beans, chocolate, and dried fruits are prone to contamination by mycotoxins. Mycotoxins can lead to various health issues in humans, such as kidney problems, liver disorders, bleeding syndromes, immune system dysfunctions, neurological conditions, and different types of cancer. These toxic substances can enter the body through skin contact, consumption, or inhalation. In developing nations, the presence of mycotoxin-contaminated food is more prevalent due to factors such as hot climate, inadequate food safety protocols, and the export of top-quality foods, in contrast to developed countries where various stages of food production are monitored. Reports suggest that approximately 500 million people in developing nations are affected by mycotoxins. The Food and Agriculture Organization has reported that mycotoxins

IntechOpen

impact about 25% of the world's crops annually, leading to approximately 1 billion metric tons of food lost each year [1, 2].

Even in wealthier countries, certain groups, such as densely populated urban areas where molds can develop and produce mycotoxins, may be vulnerable to mycotoxin exposure. Around a quarter of the world's crops are affected by mycotoxins. It is impossible to completely eliminate mycotoxins because they are a natural food contaminant, and their presence in food products is inevitable. Regulations worldwide set maximum permissible levels for mycotoxins due to their toxicity, and it is necessary to monitor their presence in various products to ensure the safety of food and protect consumers. As a result, different detection tools have been developed to detect even small amounts of toxins in food. Established methods such as

Detection method	**Advantages**	**Disadvantages**
Old methods		
1. TLC (thin layer chromatography)	Low cost, simple, and straightforward, requires minimal equipment	Low sensitivity, time-consuming, requires skilled personnel for interpretation
2. HPLC (high-performance liquid chromatography)	High resolution and specificity, well-established, can analyze multiple mycotoxins simultaneously	Expensive setup, requires skilled analysts, and longer analysis times compared to some newer method
3. LC-MS/MS (liquid chromatography-mass spectrometry)	Extremely sensitive and specific, can simultaneously analyze multiple mycotoxins, minimal sample preparation	High cost and complexity, requires skilled technicians, maintenance intensive
4. ELISA (enzyme-linked immunosorbent)	Relatively quick, user-friendly, good sensitivity for specific mycotoxins	Limited range of mycotoxins, potential for cross-reactivity, may require expensive reagents
5. Biosensors	Rapid and real-time results, portable and easy to use, potential for field testing	Developmental stage for many, can be less reliable, limited to specific mycotoxins
Novel methods		
1. Fluorescent polarization	Sensitive and allows for real-time-monitoring, minimal sample preparation needed, can analyze complex matrice	Limited to specific analytes, calibration, and interference issues, requires specialized equipment
2. Electronic nose	Rapid analysis and real-time results, non-destructive and portable, can detect a range of volatile compounds	May lack specificity, performance can vary with environmental conditions, requires complex data analysis and pattern recognition
3. Aggregation-induced emission (AIE)	Highly sensitive to low concentration, potential for specific and selective detection, simple operation, and quick response	Limited development for widespread applications requires careful design of AIE materials, environmental stability issues for some AIE compounds
4. Molecularly imprinted polymers (MIPs)	High selectivity for target compounds, stable and reusable, can be tailored to specific applications	Time-consuming synthesis process may require optimization for matrix effects, potential issues with the leaching of the polymer matrix

Table 1.
Mycotoxin detection methods in the past and present decades.

chromatography techniques, for example, high-performance liquid chromatography (HPLC) with fluorescence detection (HPLC-FLD), liquid chromatography-tandem mass spectrometry (LC-MS/MS), and gas chromatography (GC) have been widely utilized and demonstrate high specificity and sensitivity. Gas chromatography is a method that separates elements in a combination based on their behavior of dividing between stationary and mobile phases. In gas chromatography, volatile compounds are divided using a gas, such as helium, as the moving phase and a high-boiling liquid absorbed on a solid as the immobile phase. The process involves the dispersion of elements between these phases because of their different properties and structures, resulting in different retention times in the column and subsequent division. However, traditional methods lack the speed of new techniques, are costly, and require large equipment and skilled operators. Enzyme-linked immunosorbent assay (ELISA) is a widely used immune-chemical-based technique for detecting mycotoxin metabolites, offering outstanding sensitivity and specificity, as well as high sample throughput. Nonetheless, ELISA is labor-intensive and slower compared to new detection methods. Therefore, point-of-care testing (POCT) has become a major focus in recent years, offering advantages such as quickness, low sample consumption, and ease of use over central lab methods. Biosensors, as a type of POCT method and immunochemical-based technique, provide an alternative to currently frequently used methods [2, 3].

This chapter provides an overview of mycotoxin detection technologies from ancient times to the present, in order to provide references for researchers and suggestions for future research directions and early warning mycotoxin detection (**Table 1**).

2. Traditional techniques

Various methods have been utilized to analyze the presence of mycotoxins in food and feed since their discovery. Chromatographic techniques, including thin layer chromatography (TLC) and high-performance liquid chromatography (HPLC), with detectors like diode array, fluorescence, and UV, are commonly used. Liquid chromatography-tandem mass spectrometry (LC-MS/MS) and gas chromatography-tandem mass spectrometry (GC-MS/MS) are popular for mycotoxin detection [4]. Immunoassay methods like enzyme-linked immunosorbent assay (ELISA) and lateral flow immunoassay (LFIA) are crucial for rapid analysis, while biosensors are also effective in identifying mycotoxins in food [2].

2.1 Chromatography methods

2.1.1 Thin layer chromatography (TLC)

TLC is a popular and cost-effective method for detecting mycotoxins, with a stationary phase on inert materials like plastic or glass and a mobile phase made up of methanol, acetonitrile, and water mixtures. It is effective for detecting mycotoxins, with fluorescent spots under UV light. While it is useful for qualitative and quantitative analysis, TLC has low sensitivity and accuracy, making quantification challenging [5]. Sample preparation and clean-up procedures are key requirements, depending on the properties of the mycotoxin. Despite its limitations, TLC remains an important tool for screening a large number of samples for mycotoxins [6].

2.1.2 Liquid chromatography (LC)

LC methods have been developed to address the limitations of TLC, allowing for the simultaneous determination of multiple mycotoxins regardless of their chemical structure. LC uses an analytical column and mobile phase to separate analytes from matrix components, making it suitable for high polarity, non-volatile, and thermally labile mycotoxins. HPLC is commonly used for mycotoxin analysis, with different adsorbents depending on the mycotoxin's physical and chemical structure. Detection methods include UV and fluorescent detectors, as well as mass spectrometry. Some toxins naturally fluoresce, while others require derivatization to enhance detection. Derivatization can be done before or after chromatographic separation. The main limitations of HPLC include portability issues and challenges related to matrix effects, sample type, and calibration. LC offers a more versatile and effective approach to mycotoxin analysis than TLC, with a wider range of detection capabilities and fewer restrictions [2]. The use of LC-MS/MS has significantly increased in the past 20 years for detecting low molecular weight contaminants and residues at trace levels. When combined with LC, MS/MS offers improved sensitivity and reliability, making it a valuable standard tool for addressing analytical challenges in food and feed safety chemical analysis, whether in research or commercial investigation [7]. LC-MS/MS delivers high selectivity and sensitivity, as well as greater certainty in identifying analytes and a broader range of matrices compared to traditional methods using conventional detectors [8]. Many mycotoxigenic fungi can produce multiple mycotoxins simultaneously, leading to potential simultaneous contamination of agricultural commodities by different mycotoxins [9, 10]. Numerous studies have confirmed that LC-MS/MS provides reliable and sensitive results for the simultaneous determination of multi-mycotoxins analysis [2, 11–14].

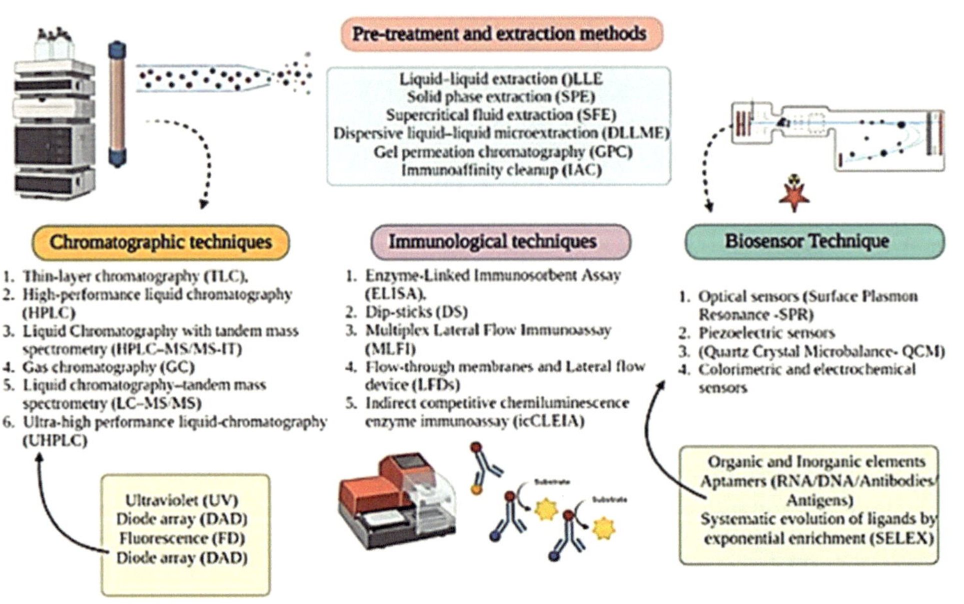

Figure 1.
Schematic representation of traditional techniques applied for the detection of mycotoxins in food matrices [18].

2.1.3 Gas chromatography (GC)

The separation in GC relies on the differential distribution of substances between the stationary and mobile phases of the column. Following the separation, volatile compounds are identified using a mass spectrometer, electron capture detector (ECD), or flame ionization detector (FID) [5]. GC is not commonly employed for mycotoxin analysis due to the low volatility and high polarity of the substances. Additionally, a derivatization step is necessary to convert them into volatile derivatives [15]. Nevertheless, the GC-MS/MS method has been utilized to detect mycotoxins in products made from milled grain [16] and wheat semolina [17].

This technique is sensitive and specific to mycotoxins, allowing for derivatization to a volatile compound suitable for gas chromatography. Challenges in mycotoxin GC analysis include column blockage, drifting responses, cross-contamination, and nonlinearity in calibration curves (**Figure 1**) [5].

3. Rapid techniques

3.1 Enzyme-linked immunosorbent assay (ELISA)

Moreover, immunochemical techniques like ELISA offer a rapid and uncomplicated screening method for on-site mycotoxin analysis; in addition to the sensitive yet intricate and expensive chromatographic methods, ELISA's design is uncomplicated, allowing for simultaneous testing of multiple samples and providing precise detection [4, 19]. It is a high-throughput assay that requires a small sample volume and involves fewer clean-up procedures compared to chromatographic methods like HPLC or TLC [5].

The test relies on the interaction of the antigen-antibody complex with chromogenic substrates, and the measurable result is obtained through spectrophotometric assessment [20]. Solcan et al. also utilized ELISA to identify AFB1 residues in chicken liver samples [21]. However, this technique has its drawbacks. Compounds with similar chemical groups can interfere with the antibodies. The occurrence of matrix effect or matrix interference in the ELISA method may result in under- or overestimation of mycotoxin concentrations in tested samples [22]. Additionally, the limited validation of ELISA restricts its application to the matrices for which it has been validated [23]. Therefore, a thorough assessment of ELISA accuracy across a wide range of food commodities is necessary [24].

3.2 Lateral flow immunoassay (LFIA)

The LFIA, also known as the immunochromatographic strip test, is an immunoassay based on a membrane and operates as a competitive method, utilizing a labeled antibody as a signal reagent [25]. During the test, the analyte is transported through capillary beds, such as pieces of porous paper, and specific recognition elements bind to moieties immobilized on the membrane surface [26]. The accuracy of LFIA primarily relies on the signal labels. Traditionally, gold nanoparticles (GNPs) are the most commonly used labels for producing visual signals [27]. In addition to nanoparticles, other materials such as magnetic nanoparticles (MNPs) [28], carbon nanoparticles (CNPs) [29], gold nanoparticles (AuNPs) [30], or quantum dots (QDs) [31] have been utilized as labels. LFIA offers numerous benefits, including its simplicity, rapid results, and cost-effectiveness, making it well-suited for large-scale on-site screening. Additionally, it eliminates the need for sample clean-up [32]. However, LFD is constrained by potential interferences and the complexity of analyzing trace analytes within the matrix [33].

3.3 Biosensors

The sensing element in biosensors is typically biological or biologically derived and is used to detect specific bio-analytes. It is integrated with a transducer to convert biological signals into electrical signals [34]. Mycotoxin detection can utilize various transducers, such as electrochemical (potentiometric, amperometric, and impedimetric), optical (surface plasmon resonance-SPR and fluorescence), and piezoelectric (quartz crystal microbalance (QCM)) [35]. Nucleic acids, peptides, enzymes, antibodies, and cells are commonly recognized materials, but other bioinspired elements like recombinant antibodies, aptamers, and molecularly imprinted polymers (MIPs) can also be employed [36]. Additionally, to enhance biosensor sensitivity, a diverse range of metal nanoparticles, carbon nanotubes (CNTs), nanofibers, and QDs are utilized for their biocompatibility, physicochemical properties, and high surface volume ratio [37]. The detection methodologies for electrochemical biosensors include potentiometric, amperometric, and impedimetric techniques [38]. A potentiometric sensor utilizes either two (working and reference) or three (working, reference, and counter) electrode systems, with changes in circuit potential between working and reference electrodes indicating a recognition event. Like potentiometric sensors, amperometric sensors also require a two- or three-electrode system. The identification of an analyte with an amperometric transducer involves analyzing the current data generated from the reduction and oxidation of immobilized electroactive species on the working surface at an appropriate potential [35]. Electrochemical impedance spectroscopy (EIS) observes changes in the interface between the electrode surface and a nanostructured platform in contact with a redox probe [39]. The primary benefits of optical biosensors are their high sensitivity and real-time analysis capabilities [40]. Commonly used methods include surface plasmon resonance (SPR) and fluorescence-based approaches such as fluorescence resonance energy transfer (FRET) [41]. In the SPR system, a thin metal film (silver or gold) is positioned between two transparent media with different refractive indices, such as a glass prism and sample solution. Changes in the refractive index of the surface layer in contact with the sensor chip are detected using the SPR method. In the FRET system, energy is transferred from an excited donor fluorophore to nearby acceptor species. The FRET system allows for the design of biunique or one-to-multiple acceptor and donor configurations, enabling simultaneous multiple mycotoxin detection [2].

The QCM transducer comprises a thin gold-plated crystal quartz with electrodes placed on it. When a molecular recognition and binding event occurs on the electrode surface, it leads to mass alteration and specific vibrations. These vibrations induce changes in the resonant frequency when an electric signal is sent by the quartz [2]. The analysis of mycotoxins at a rapid pace offers several shared benefits, such as quickness, affordability, simplicity, and user-friendliness [24]. Key factors to consider are the ability to be portable and the capability to detect multiple toxins. Mobility is also crucial due to the increasing need for on-site testing, which could occur, for instance, at the location of food production. This approach yields results relatively swiftly, as there is no requirement to ship samples for analysis in laboratories, thus preventing delays in the food production process. The detection of multiple toxins removes the necessity for conducting numerous individual tests for a single sample batch [2]. However, these methods have some main limitations, including interference from the sample matrix, cross-reactivity of antibodies, and the need for validation of matrices (**Figures 2** and **3**) [2, 5].

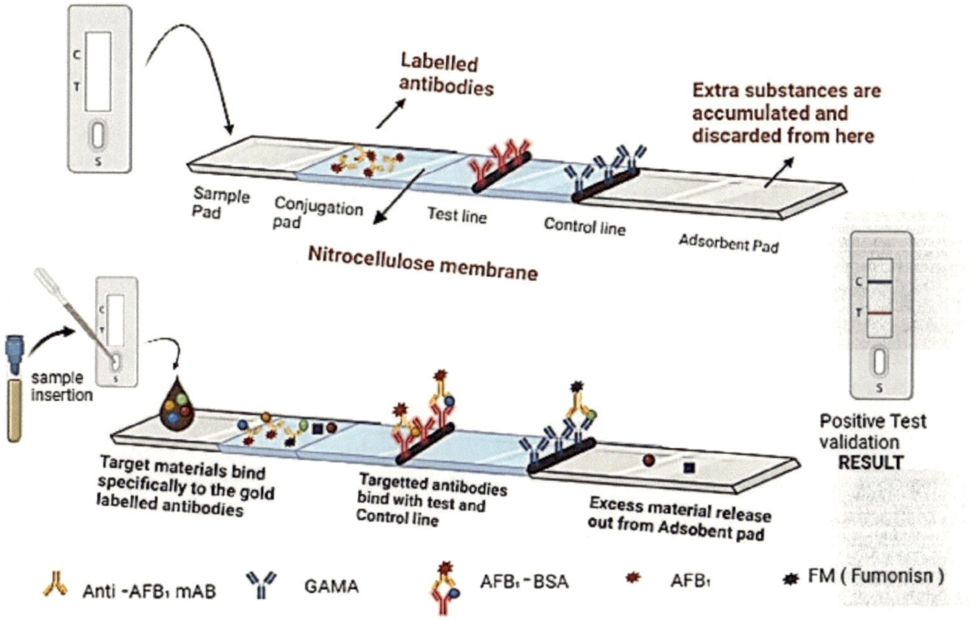

Figure 2.
Schematic representation of rapid techniques applied for the detection of mycotoxins in food matrices [42].

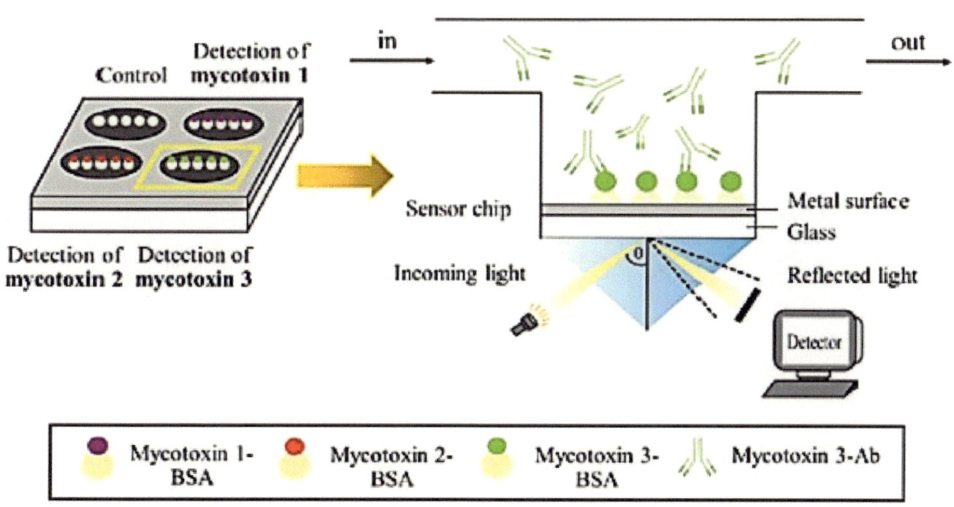

Figure 3.
Schematic diagram of an SPR immunosensor chip for multiple (rapid techniques) mycotoxin detection [43].

4. Novel techniques

Apart from the standard techniques mentioned earlier, there are various other approaches that have been created that could be valuable for detecting mycotoxins. However, these techniques are not widely employed beyond research settings and have limited practicality. Additionally, they need to undergo further confirmation and validation by reputable organizations like the Association of Official Analytical Chemists (AOAC), the International Organization for Standardization (ISO), or the European Standardization Committee (CEN) [2, 15].

4.1 Electronic nose

The electronic nose (e-nose) consists of various non-specific chemical detectors that capture a wide range of volatile organic compounds (VOCs) and identify qualitative patterns related to toxigenic fungi. Once a fingerprint is created, detecting the odor provides preliminary information about the types of metabolites produced by a system that recognizes these patterns [44]. The e-nose technology for identifying fungal infections focuses on detecting specific VOCs linked to fungal growth on cereal grains. The growth and biochemical behavior of mycotoxigenic fungal species results in chemical changes in VOC composition, establishing a relationship between VOCs and mycotoxin levels in food [45]. The e-nose has successfully detected ochratoxin A (OTA) dry-cured meat [46], AFs and fumonisins in maize [45], and deoxynivalenol (DON) in wheat bran and durum wheat [47]. To enable broad application of e-nose in mycotoxin detection, it is essential to optimize the quantification of low mycotoxin levels in food samples. Additionally, the majority of mycotoxins are non-volatile organic compounds, posing a challenge for e-nose detection [15].

4.2 Fluorescent polarization

The fluorescent polarization (FP) immunoassay relies on the competition between the analyte and the tracer for specific sites on the antibody. When the tracer binds to the antibody, it influences the rotation of the tracer molecule, resulting in an

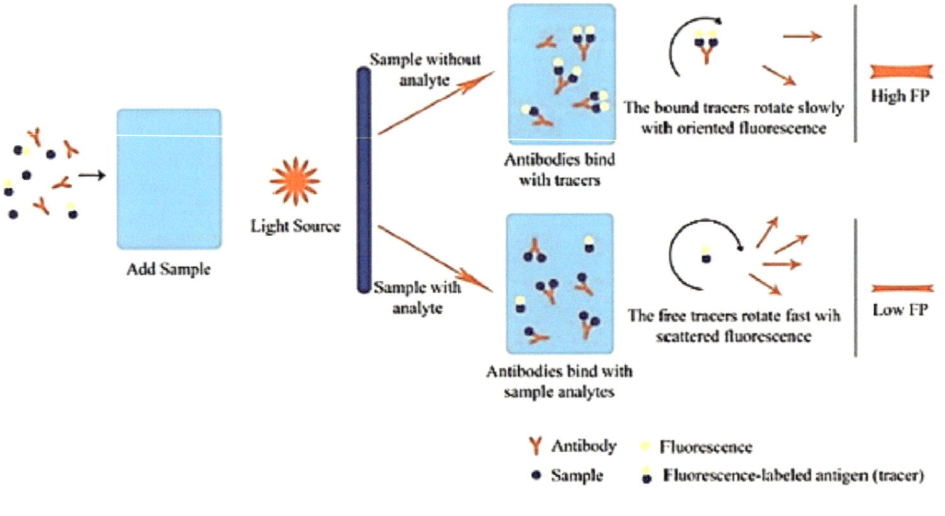

Figure 4.
Schematic for fluorescent polarization mycotoxin detection [51].

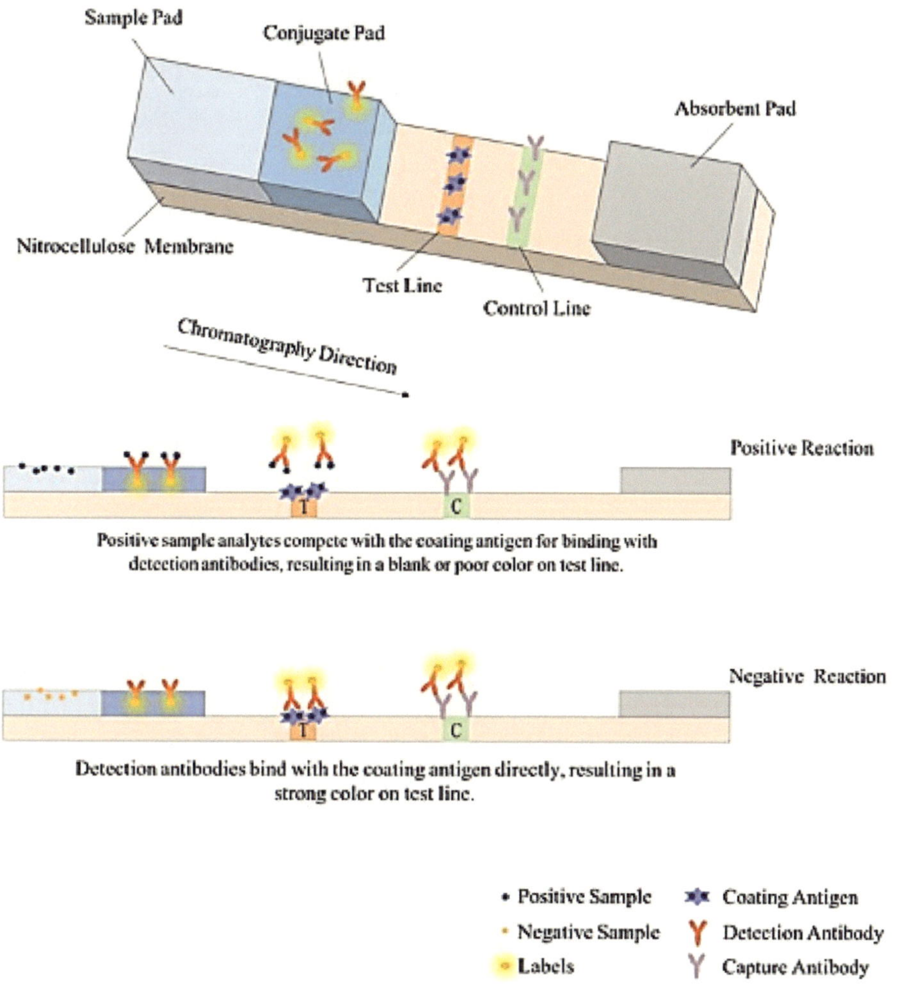

Figure 5.
Schematic for immunochromatographic assay for nitrofurans detection [51].

increase in the fluorescence polarization value. The polarization value is inversely proportional to the concentration of the analyte, as the amount of bound tracer decreases with the amount of free analyte in the sample [48]. Unlike ELISA, the FP technique eliminates the need for time-consuming pre-analytical steps such as washing multiple times or separating free from antibody-bound analyte. The FP immunoassay has been utilized to detect different mycotoxins in food items, such as zearalenone (ZEA) in corn [49], DON in wheat products, AFB1 in corn, and OTA in rice [50], AFB1 in maize, and OTA in rice. However, this method's sensitivity and accuracy are not as high as those of HPLC, likely because of the cross-reactivity of antibodies with other fungal metabolites and components in the food matrix (**Figures 4** and 5) [15].

4.3 The emission induced by aggregation

Aggregation-induced emission (AIE) is when fluorescent dyes emit a faint glow in a diluted solution but shine brightly when aggregated [2]. This enhanced fluorescence

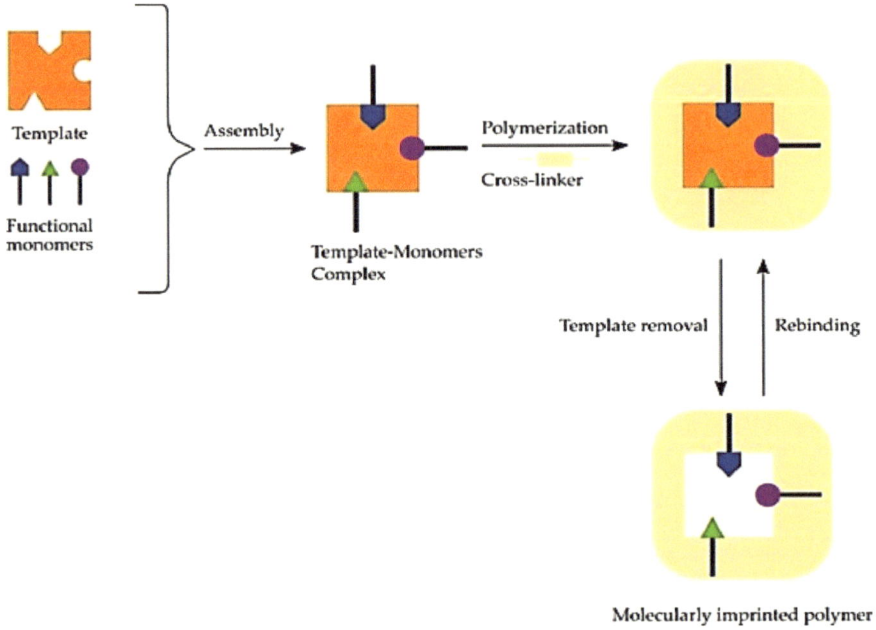

Figure 6.
Scheme of molecularly imprinted polymer preparation [2].

is due to limited intramolecular rotations. Dyes like 9,10-distyrylanthracene (DSA), silacyclopentadiene (silole), tetraphenylethene (TPE), and their derivatives show high fluorescence in aggregated states. AIE dye-based aptasensors are effective for detecting OTA in wine and coffee, as well as AFB1 in peanut oil and broad bean sauce.

4.4 Molecularly imprinted polymers

Molecularly imprinted polymers (MIPs) mimic natural recognition agents like antibodies and biological receptors, with specificity comparable to antibody-antigen interactions. The process involves creating cross-linked polymers by copolymerizing functional monomers and a cross-linker in the presence of a template analyte [52]. MIPs offer high selectivity and affinity for the target molecule, along with resistance to temperature, pressure, bases, acids, metal ions, and solvents. They are cost-effective to synthesize, have long-term storage capabilities, and can retain recognition abilities for years at room temperature [53]. MIPs have been successfully used to detect mycotoxins like AFB1 in wheat, OTA in beer and wine, and ZEA in cereals, showing promise for further advancements in mycotoxin detection (**Figure 6**) [2].

5. Conclusion

The evolution from traditional to modern methods of mycotoxin detection reflects a broader trend in scientific research toward greater accuracy and efficiency. While traditional methods laid the groundwork for understanding mycotoxins, contemporary techniques offer the tools necessary to address the challenges of food safety in an increasingly complex world. As research continues to advance, the ongoing development of innovative detection methods will be crucial in safeguarding public health and ensuring the safety of our food supply.

Conflict of interest

The author declares no conflict of interest.

Author details

Leila Faeli
Department of Parasitology and Mycology, School of Medicine, Baqiyatallah University of Medical Sciences, Tehran, Iran

*Address all correspondence to: faeli.leila@gmail.com

References

[1] Liew W-P-P, Mohd-Redzwan S. Mycotoxin: Its impact on gut health and microbiota. Frontiers in Cellular and Infection Microbiology. 2018;**8**:60

[2] Janik E, Niemcewicz M, Podogrocki M, Ceremuga M, Gorniak L, Stela M, et al. The existing methods and novel approaches in mycotoxins' detection. Molecules. 2021;**26**(13):3981

[3] Szelenberger R, Cichoń N, Zajaczkowski W, Bijak M. Application of biosensors for the detection of mycotoxins for the improvement of food safety. Toxins. 2024;**16**(6):249

[4] Urusov A, Zherdev A, Dzantiev B. Immunochemical methods of mycotoxin analysis. Applied Biochemistry and Microbiology. 2010;**46**:253-266

[5] Singh J, Mehta A. Rapid and sensitive detection of mycotoxins by advanced and emerging analytical methods: A review. Food Science & Nutrition. 2020;**8**(5):2183-2204

[6] Yang J, Li J, Jiang Y, Duan X, Qu H, Yang B, et al. Natural occurrence, analysis, and prevention of mycotoxins in fruits and their processed products. Critical Reviews in Food Science and Nutrition. 2014;**54**(1):64-83

[7] Malachová A, Stránská M, Václavíková M, Elliott CT, Black C, Meneely J, et al. Advanced LC–MS-based methods to study the co-occurrence and metabolization of multiple mycotoxins in cereals and cereal-based food. Analytical and Bioanalytical Chemistry. 2018;**410**:801-825

[8] Pascale M, De Girolamo A, Lippolis V, Stroka J, Mol HG, Lattanzio VM. Performance evaluation of LC-MS methods for multimycotoxin determination. Journal of AOAC International. 2019;**102**(6):1708-1720

[9] Shi H, Li S, Bai Y, Prates LL, Lei Y, Yu P. Mycotoxin contamination of food and feed in China: Occurrence, detection techniques, toxicological effects and advances in mitigation technologies. Food Control. 2018;**91**:202-215

[10] Smith M-C, Madec S, Coton E, Hymery N. Natural co-occurrence of mycotoxins in foods and feeds and their in vitro combined toxicological effects. Toxins. 2016;**8**(4):94

[11] Bessaire T, Mujahid C, Mottier P, Desmarchelier A. Multiple mycotoxins determination in food by LC-MS/MS: An international collaborative study. Toxins. 2019;**11**(11):658

[12] Flores-Flores ME, González-Peñas E. An LC–MS/MS method for multi-mycotoxin quantification in cow milk. Food Chemistry. 2017;**218**:378-385

[13] Abdallah MF, Girgin G, Baydar T, Krska R, Sulyok M. Occurrence of multiple mycotoxins and other fungal metabolites in animal feed and maize samples from Egypt using LC-MS/MS. Journal of the Science of Food and Agriculture. 2017;**97**(13):4419-4428

[14] Al-Taher F, Banaszewski K, Jackson L, Zweigenbaum J, Ryu D, Cappozzo J. Rapid method for the determination of multiple mycotoxins in wines and beers by LC-MS/MS using a stable isotope dilution assay. Journal of Agricultural and Food Chemistry. 2013;**61**(10):2378-2384

[15] Alshannaq A, Yu J-H. Occurrence, toxicity, and analysis of major

mycotoxins in food. International Journal of Environmental Research and Public Health. 2017;**14**(6):632

[16] Rodríguez-Carrasco Y, Moltó JC, Berrada H, Mañes J. A survey of trichothecenes, zearalenone and patulin in milled grain-based products using GC–MS/MS. Food Chemistry. 2014;**146**:212-219

[17] Rodríguez-Carrasco Y, Berrada H, Font G, Mañes J. Multi-mycotoxin analysis in wheat semolina using an acetonitrile-based extraction procedure and gas chromatography–tandem mass spectrometry. Journal of Chromatography. A. 2012;**1270**:28-40

[18] Pushparaj K, Meyyazhagan A, Pappuswamy M, Mousavi Khaneghah A, Liu WC, Balasubramanian B. Occurrence, identification, and decontamination of potential mycotoxins in fruits and fruit by-products. Food Frontiers. 2023;**4**(1):32-46

[19] Oplatowska-Stachowiak M, Reiring C, Sajic N, Haasnoot W, Brabet C, Campbell K, et al. Development and in-house validation of a rapid and simple to use ELISA for the detection and measurement of the mycotoxin sterigmatocystin. Analytical and Bioanalytical Chemistry. 2018;**410**:3017-3023

[20] Li P, Zhang Q, Zhang W. Immunoassays for aflatoxins. TrAC, Trends in Analytical Chemistry. 2009;**28**(9):1115-1126

[21] Solcan C, Gogu M, Floristean V, Oprisan B, Solcan G. The hepatoprotective effect of sea buckthorn (*Hippophae rhamnoides*) berries on induced aflatoxin B1 poisoning in chickens. Poultry Science. 2013;**92**(4):966-974

[22] Thway T, Salimi-Moosavi H. Evaluating the impact of matrix effects on biomarker assay sensitivity. Bioanalysis. 2014;**6**(8):1081-1091

[23] Omar SS, Haddad MA, Parisi S. Validation of HPLC and Enzyme-Linked Immunosorbent Assay (ELISA) techniques for detection and quantification of aflatoxins in different food samples. Food. 2020;**9**(5):661

[24] Zheng MZ, Richard JL, Binder J. A review of rapid methods for the analysis of mycotoxins. Mycopathologia. 2006;**161**(5):261-273

[25] Song S, Liu N, Zhao Z, Njumbe Ediage E, Wu S, Sun C, et al. Multiplex lateral flow immunoassay for mycotoxin determination. Analytical Chemistry. 2014;**86**(10):4995-5001

[26] Anfossi L, Baggiani C, Giovannoli C, D'Arco G, Giraudi G. Lateral-flow immunoassays for mycotoxins and phycotoxins: A review. Analytical and Bioanalytical Chemistry. 2013;**405**:467-480

[27] Li R, Meng C, Wen Y, Fu W, He P. Fluorometric lateral flow immunoassay for simultaneous determination of three mycotoxins (aflatoxin B 1, zearalenone and deoxynivalenol) using quantum dot microbeads. Microchimica Acta. 2019;**186**:1-9

[28] Wang Y, Xu H, Wei M, Gu H, Xu Q, Zhu W. Study of superparamagnetic nanoparticles as labels in the quantitative lateral flow immunoassay. Materials Science and Engineering: C. 2009;**29**(3):714-718

[29] Zhang X, Yu X, Wen K, Li C, Mujtaba Mari G, Jiang H, et al. Multiplex lateral flow immunoassays based on amorphous carbon nanoparticles for detecting three fusarium mycotoxins in maize. Journal

of Agricultural and Food Chemistry. 2017;**65**(36):8063-8071

[30] Li Y, Liu L, Kuang H, Xu C. Visible and eco-friendly immunoassays for the detection of cyclopiazonic acid in maize and rice. Journal of Food Science. 2020;**85**(1):105-113

[31] Anfossi L, Di Nardo F, Cavalera S, Giovannoli C, Spano G, Speranskaya ES, et al. A lateral flow immunoassay for straightforward determination of fumonisin mycotoxins based on the quenching of the fluorescence of CdSe/ZnS quantum dots by gold and silver nanoparticles. Microchimica Acta. 2018;**185**:1-10

[32] Liu Z, Hua Q, Wang J, Liang Z, Li J, Wu J, et al. A smartphone-based dual detection mode device integrated with two lateral flow immunoassays for multiplex mycotoxins in cereals. Biosensors and Bioelectronics. 2020;**158**:112178

[33] Krska R, Molinelli A. Rapid test strips for analysis of mycotoxins in food and feed. Analytical and Bioanalytical Chemistry. 2009;**393**:67-71

[34] Perumal V, Hashim U. Advances in biosensors: Principle, architecture and applications. Journal of Applied Biomedicine. 2014;**12**(1):1-15

[35] Oliveira IS, da Silva Junior AG, de Andrade CAS, Oliveira MDL. Biosensors for early detection of fungi spoilage and toxigenic and mycotoxins in food. Current Opinion in Food Science. 2019;**29**:64-79

[36] Malekzad H, Sahandi Zangabad P, Mirshekari H, Karimi M, Hamblin MR. Noble metal nanoparticles in biosensors: Recent studies and applications. Nanotechnology Reviews. 2017;**6**(3):301-329

[37] Doria G, Conde J, Veigas B, Giestas L, Almeida C, Assunção M, et al. Noble metal nanoparticles for biosensing applications. Sensors. 2012;**12**(2):1657-1687

[38] Fernández H, Arévalo FJ, Granero AM, Robledo SN, Diaz Nieto CH, Riberi WI, et al. Electrochemical biosensors for the determination of toxic substances related to food safety developed in South America: Mycotoxins and herbicides. Chem. 2017;**5**(3):23

[39] Chai C, Oh S-W. Electrochemical impedimetric biosensors for food safety. Food Science and Biotechnology. 2020;**29**:879-887

[40] Chen C, Wang J. Optical biosensors: An exhaustive and comprehensive review. The Analyst. 2020;**145**(5):1605-1628

[41] LaVasseur C, Neukam S, Kartika T, Bannow BS, Shatzel J, DeLoughery TG. Hormonal therapies and venous thrombosis: Considerations for prevention and management. Research and Practice in Thrombosis and Haemostasis. 2022;**6**(6):e12763

[42] Jubeen F, Batool A, Naz I, Sehar S, Sadia H, Hayat A, et al. Mycotoxins detection in food using advanced, sensitive and robust electrochemical platform of sensors: A review. Sensors and Actuators A: Physical. 2024;**367**:115045

[43] Adunphatcharaphon S, Elliott CT, Sooksimuang T, Charlermroj R, Petchkongkaew A, Karoonuthaisiri N. The evolution of multiplex detection of mycotoxins using immunoassay platform technologies. Journal of Hazardous Materials. 2022;**432**:128706

[44] Leggieri MC, Mazzoni M, Fodil S, Moschini M, Bertuzzi T, Prandini A,

et al. An electronic nose supported by an artificial neural network for the rapid detection of aflatoxin B1 and fumonisins in maize. Food Control. 2021;**123**:107722

[45] Ottoboni M, Pinotti L, Tretola M, Giromini C, Fusi E, Rebucci R, et al. Combining E-nose and lateral flow immunoassays (LFIAs) for rapid occurrence/co-occurrence aflatoxin and fumonisin detection in maize. Toxins. 2018;**10**(10):416

[46] Lippolis V, Ferrara M, Cervellieri S, Damascelli A, Epifani F, Pascale M, et al. Rapid prediction of ochratoxin A-producing strains of Penicillium on dry-cured meat by MOS-based electronic nose. International Journal of Food Microbiology. 2016;**218**:71-77

[47] Lippolis V, Pascale M, Cervellieri S, Damascelli A, Visconti A. Screening of deoxynivalenol contamination in durum wheat by MOS-based electronic nose and identification of the relevant pattern of volatile compounds. Food Control. 2014;**37**:263-271

[48] Valenzano S, Lippolis V, Pascale M, De Marco A, Maragos CM, Suman M, et al. Determination of deoxynivalenol in wheat bran and whole-wheat flour by fluorescence polarization immunoassay. Food Analytical Methods. 2014;**7**:806-813

[49] Zhang X, Eremin SA, Wen K, Yu X, Li C, Ke Y, et al. Fluorescence polarization immunoassay based on a new monoclonal antibody for the detection of the zearalenone class of mycotoxins in maize. Journal of Agricultural and Food Chemistry. 2017;**65**(10):2240-2247

[50] Lippolis V, Pascale M, Visconti A. Optimization of a fluorescence polarization immunoassay for rapid quantification of deoxynivalenol in durum wheat–based products. Journal of Food Protection. 2006;**69**(11):2712-2719

[51] Wu W, Yang S, Liu J, Mi J, Dou L, Pan Y, et al. Progress in immunoassays for nitrofurans detection. Food and Agricultural Immunology. 2020;**31**(1):907-926

[52] Vasapollo G, Sole RD, Mergola L, Lazzoi MR, Scardino A, Scorrano S, et al. Molecularly imprinted polymers: Present and future prospective. International Journal of Molecular Sciences. 2011;**12**(9):5908-5945

[53] Krska R, Welzig E, Berthiller F, Molinelli A, Mizaikoff B. Advances in the analysis of mycotoxins and its quality assurance. Food Additives and Contaminants. 2005;**22**(4):345-353

Chapter 4

Mycotoxins and Mitigation Plan

Mehdi Fathollahi, Razieh Noroozi, Parisa Shavali-gilani and Ebrahim Molaee-aghaee

Abstract

The best strategy to deal with mycotoxins is to prevent their production and implement Good Agricultural Practices in their cultivation, storage, and transport stages throughout the food chain. However, in many cases, their occurrence in foodstuffs such as different grains and also animal-based foods like meat and milk by their contaminated feed threatens food safety and consumer health. Therefore, the most effective way is to inactivate and prevent the growth of the mycotoxin-producing fungi, followed by the degradation of mycotoxins without using chemicals as much as possible to maintain their nutritional value. Some thermal and non-thermal processes and a combination of them in the food industry may be useful strategies to reduce the risks raised by a variety of fungi like *Aspergillus, Penicillium*, etc., and their exerted mycotoxins like aflatoxins, ochratoxins, etc. in food products.

Keywords: mycotoxin, prevention, detoxification, non-thermal processes, food safety

1. Introduction

Molds are ubiquitous and can occur in pre-harvest periods with contributing factors and stress conditions such as drought, flooding, insect infestation and late harvest) and after harvesting, including transportation and storage (contributing factors: insufficient drying, hot and humid environment), causing food contamination. Among the factors affecting the amount of food contamination with molds and mycotoxin production include Geographical location, processes performed on food and environmental factors including temperature, water activity and pH, damage to the product by insects and product density affect the growth of fungi and mycotoxin production [1].

1.1 The natural presence of mycotoxins

Cereals are one of the main ingredients in the diet of humans and animals that are contaminated by mycotoxin-producing molds. About 400 different types of mycotoxins have been identified, mainly produced by molds of the genera *Aspergillus, Penicillium, Fusarium* and *Trichotecium*. Their most important mycotoxins include aflatoxin B1, ochratoxin A, zearalenone, deoxynivalenol, fumonisin B1 and toxin T-2. The fungi responsible for producing these mycotoxins are often endophytes that infect living plant tissues and create colonies; the accumulation of mycotoxins in plant tissues may sometimes be associated with the development of disease symptoms in the plant. The chemical structure of the main mycotoxins is shown in **Figure 1** [2, 3].

IntechOpen

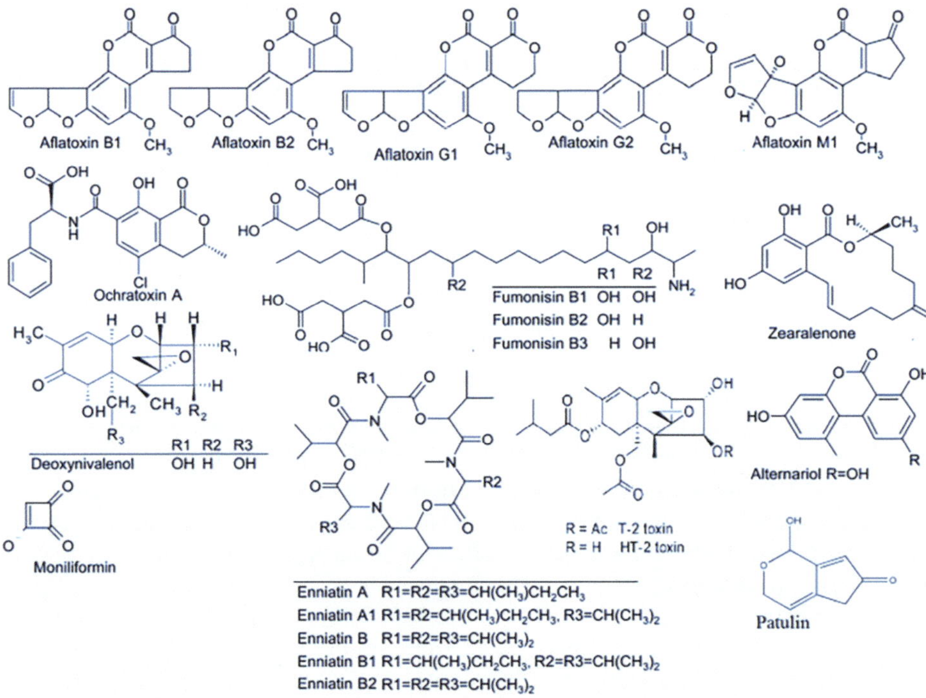

Figure 1.
Chemical structures of major mycotoxins [2].

It is practically impossible to prevent the growth and development of fungi and the production of mycotoxins. But there are different techniques to reduce food contamination, which generally include physical, chemical and biological methods [4].

1.2 Toxic effects of mycotoxins on health

Mycotoxins are silent killers and their effects may go undetected for a long time, especially if they are regularly exposed. When consumed or inhaled, mycotoxins cause a variety of metabolic disorders in humans and animals, including negative effects on the immune system, malignancies, allergies, abortion, and, in rare cases, the death of the host [5].

Mycotoxins are involved in causing liver cancer, growth disorder, acute toxicity (aflatoxin), esophageal cancer and neural tube defects (NTDS) (fumonisins) and gastroenteritis (deoxynivalenol (DON)) and kidney disease (ochratoxin A (OTA)) [6].

In animals, mycotoxins can cause chronic diseases, reproductive problems, and sudden death. For example, aflatoxins can cause liver damage or cancer, reduce milk and egg production in livestock and poultry, and suppress the immune system [7].

1.3 Strategies to prevent the production of mycotoxins in food

With three prevention processes, before and after harvest, we can prevent the contamination of products with fungi or reduce the production of mycotoxins.

Primary prevention is related to activities that aim to keep the environment unfavorable for the growth of fungi, such as

- Manage and set up good hygiene programs when harvesting crops.
- Reducing the humidity of plant seeds during harvesting and storage with appropriate methods.
- Keeping products at low temperatures.
- Use of approved fungicides to control and eliminate fungi.
- Use approved insecticides to prevent insect infestation.
- Secondary prevention occurs when fungi pass the primary prevention process and product contamination with fungi has occurred.
- Re-drying the product.
- Removal of seeds infected with fungus.
- Inactivation of produced mycotoxins.
- Creating conditions that do not cause fungus to grow [8].
- The third type of prevention is done when the crop is heavily contaminated with fungi.
- Destruction of products infected with fungi.
- Minimize or eliminate mycotoxins [9].

2. Strategies to reduce mycotoxins in food

2.1 Physical methods

2.1.1 Mechanical separation

The physical separation of damaged products from healthy products reduces the production of aflatoxin from 27–97% [10].

2.1.1.1 Sorting

It is done by manual, mechanical, photoelectric methods, or a combination of these. The efficiency of the electric method is more than the others so it reduces 70% of aflatoxin [11].

2.1.1.2 Separation based on density

Contamination of cereal grains with mycotoxins causes different physical properties from healthy grains, which separates healthy from unhealthy seeds. In this method, solutions such as sucrose, sodium chloride, hydrogen peroxide or strong airflow are used. Separation of seeds contaminated with aflatoxin by hydrogen peroxide solution and contaminated with zearalenone by air pressure in another study reduces mycotoxins [4].

2.2 Thermal process

Although mycotoxins are heat-resistant molecules, it has been shown that 50–80% of mycotoxins are destroyed in the preparation of traditional foods (cooking, frying) at a temperature of more than 1000°C. In addition, the temperature between 150 and 2000°C causes a drop of 70% in aflatoxin (AFB1) [12].

The melting point of all types of aflatoxins is between 230 and 299°C. Therefore, aflatoxin is difficult to destroy by heat using methods such as boiling, autoclaving, and frying. So 20% of aflatoxin B1 is destroyed at a temperature of 160°C for 30 minutes. It is noteworthy that the thermal process of destroying aflatoxin in wet products destroys more aflatoxin than in dry products. The reason for this is the opening of the ring. Lactone is the result of hydrolytic processes, decomposition reactions and decarboxylation process. In general, temperature and time play an important role in the thermal process of reducing mycotoxins, and studies have shown that aflatoxin degradation does not occur at temperatures below 60°C. However, at low pH at 40°C, aflatoxins B1 and G1 are destroyed. A temperature of 120°C has reduced aflatoxin by 8–20% in juices. Probably the most thermal resistance among mycotoxins is related to ochratoxin A. The thermal stability of ochratoxin A is different in different studies, such that autoclave heat in one study caused a 10% decrease and in another study caused an 89% decrease in this mycotoxin. One of the important factors in the heat stability of this mycotoxin is the moisture content of the substrate. Mycotoxins patulin, zearlenone and penicillin acid are also resistant to heat. But their stability depends on the pH of the substrate so their thermal stability increases at low pH. In the case of patulin, autoclaving heat for 120 minutes destroys 80% of this mycotoxin. Takes. Finally, the degree of degradability of mycotoxins by heat has not been confirmed. Finally, the degree of degradability of mycotoxins by heat has not been specifically confirmed. The degree of their degradation depends on factors such as temperature, time, pH, humidity and mycotoxin concentration [13].

Since temperature and humidity are two essential variables in the growth of fungi and mycotoxins, storage in controlled environments such as packaging and warehouses with proper temperature, ventilation and humidity control prevents the growth of fungi and the accumulation of mycotoxins. Product loss in underdeveloped countries is between 20 and 50% due to incorrect storage methods [14].

2.3 Irradiation

There are two types of radiation. There are ionizing (X-rays, ultraviolet rays, rays of gamma and electron beams) and non-ionizing radiations (Radio waves, microwave waves, infrared waves and visible light waves). Non-ionizing radiation with thermal methods destroys mycotoxins, and since it was explained earlier about thermal methods, we will focus on ionizing radiation.

2.4 Gamma rays

It plays an important role in the destruction of aflatoxin, and 5–10 kg radiation of this radiation destroys it. It should be noted that this radiation is not suitable for foods with high lipid and vitamin content [15].

Irradiation in fruit juice reduces zearalenone, but irradiation of more than 10 kg reduces quality. The results of a study showed that the use of gamma rays at a rate of 5 kg reduces ochratoxin A by 93% [16].

In another study, the use of gamma rays at a rate of 10 kg on peanuts increases the storage time of the product at ambient temperature without mycotoxin being produced [17].

2.5 Electron beam irradiation (EBI)

The formation of the electron beam is done through the production of electrons by a cathode using electric current in vacuum conditions, which is known as a sterilization method. The energy of electrons reduces the microbial load by breaking molecular bonds and forming free radicals. Electron beams reduced the growth of *Penicillium, Aspergillus* and *Fusarium fungi* in raw corn, and 16 kg of this radiation destroyed 91.56% of ochratoxin A and 72.29% of zearlenone [18].

2.6 Ultraviolet ray

Ultraviolet rays easily pass through liquids, but there are limitations in the case of solids. The average doses of ultraviolet radiation of 200 and 400 microvolts per cubic centimeter in peanut oil without any adverse effect on its physicochemical and sensory properties cause a loss of 79 and 85%, respectively [15].

Finally, it should be said that various studies have reported the effects of UV radiation on mycotoxins in food. In a study, UV radiation caused a 90% decrease in aflatoxin M1 with the presence of 0.5% peroxide. And 2–5 megarads of this radiation caused a 90% decrease in aflatoxin in grains [19].

2.7 X-ray

X-rays are a better alternative than gamma rays for cold pasteurization, which provides food safety with minimal impact on quality. It also has a high penetration power (30–40 cm) in food and is also used to disinfect food [20].

2.8 Pulsed light

Technology that uses short and high-intensity flashes of ultraviolet, visible and infrared rays. In a study, Abu Agla and colleagues showed a 91% reduction of aflatoxin by pulsed light, which was accompanied by slight changes in the color of peanut kernels but did not affect its chemical characteristics [21].

2.9 Pulsed electric field

A method that uses high voltage (20–80 kV/cm) for 1 second affects the membrane of the microorganism and causes its destruction [22].

2.10 Cold plasma (CP)

Plasma is a term for the fourth state of matter, which is mostly composed of photons, ions and free radicals such as active species of oxygen and nitrogen, each of which has specific physical and chemical properties. By using low-pressure cold plasma, researchers were able to detoxify up to 50% of aflatoxins on the surface of

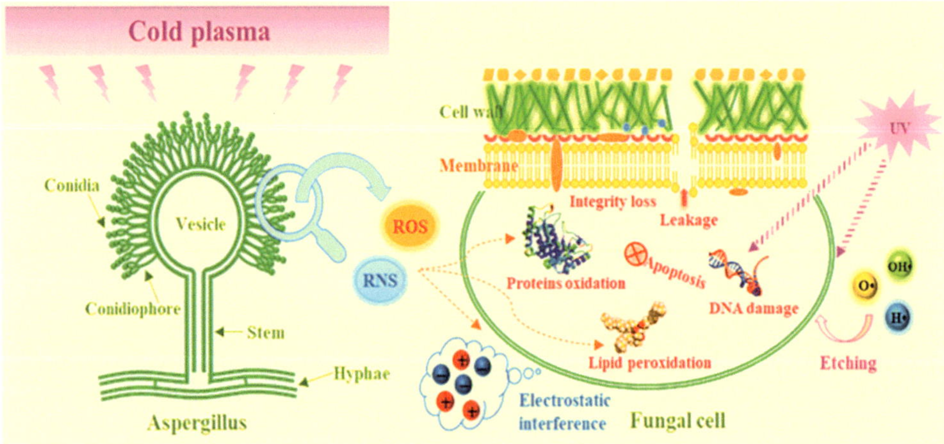

Figure 2.
How to destroy aflatoxin in cold plasma method [24].

nuts. However, this approach should be used with caution due to the lack of information on the possible creation of hazardous chemicals [23].

In a study, it was found that the use of oxygen plasma for 90 seconds in hazelnuts reduced *Aspergillus flavus* and *Aspergillus parasiticus* by nearly 100%, and the amount of aflatoxin decreased to 95% (**Figure 2**) [24].

2.11 High-pressure process (HPP)

The process of inactivating the spores of microorganisms, which by affecting the membrane, causes its integrity to be lost and causes the spores to be inactivated. This method has the least effect on the taste and organoleptic characteristics of food. Therefore, it is a suitable method to prevent the growth of food pathogens [25].

2.12 Chemical methods

There are various chemical methods for neutralizing mycotoxins in food, which cause decomposition and reduce absorption from the gut by binding to mycotoxins. Many chemicals effective in eliminating mycotoxins cannot be used because these substances themselves are toxic [26].

2.12.1 Chitosan

Chitosan is a linear polymer that inhibits microorganisms. Chitosan is the second most abundant carbohydrate in nature after cellulose. The biocompatibility and antimicrobial properties of chitosan make it a promising agent for food preservation [27].

In a study, the use of chitosan reduced the production of mycotoxins aflatoxin and doxynivalenone [28] in wheat and corn seeds [29].

2.12.2 Ozone

Ozone is a strong oxidizer that does not leave any dangerous substances after use [30, 31]. In addition to being used to sterilize grains, vegetables and fruits, ozone is also used to detoxify mycotoxins. Since aflatoxins, especially AFB1 and AFG1, have a double bond at the C8-C9 carbons in their structure, Agriopoulo et al. found that ozone gas effectively destroys them because of this double bond [32].

Studies have shown that AFG1 is the most sensitive type of aflatoxin. The positive effects of ozonation have been successfully shown in previous studies to reduce AFB1 in crops such as wheat, corn, peanuts, and red pepper. And the hepatotoxicity and renal toxicity of aflatoxin is significantly reduced [15].

In Lu et al.'s study, the amount of ozone with a concentration of 90 mg/l was used for 40 minutes on AFB1 infected corns at humidity levels of 13.47 and 20.37. The results showed a decrease in the amount of aflatoxin by 88.1 and 72.4, respectively. It can be said that the lower moisture content caused a greater effect of ozone on AFB1 [33].

Other studies have shown that ozonation of corn contaminated with AFB1 removes 90% of aflatoxin. However, it has reduced the protein content by 3.2% and changed the fatty acid profile [15].

2.12.3 Use of organic acids

Studies have shown that soaking rice, soy and pepper in organic acids has been effective in breaking down and reducing aflatoxin. For example, the use of citric acid reduces 97% of AFB1 after 96 hours at room temperature, and if exposed to heat for 20 minutes, 98% of AFB1 is destroyed. The amount of aflatoxin degradation depends on temperature, time, humidity and acid concentration [15].

In a study, Rastgar et al. found that roasting pistachio nuts with lemon juice at 120 C° reduced the amount of aflatoxin by 50.2% [34].

2.12.4 Use of alkaline substances

Aflatoxin is very unstable under alkaline conditions and the first step in the decomposition of aflatoxin is the opening of the lactone ring. Ammonium has been used many times by researchers concerning aflatoxin. And the use of gaseous ammonium or ammonium hydroxide has reduced aflatoxin by 99%. Ammonia can also be used to neutralize aflatoxin. One of the advantages of using ammonia is that it is cheap and can be used in the field, but one of its disadvantages is the effect on nutritional properties and safety problems. The noteworthy point is that ammonia is effective on mycotoxins such as aflatoxin that have a lactone ring [35].

In a study, ammonia vapor was used to decontaminate wheat grains from deoxynivalenol [28] at a temperature of 90°C for 2 hours, which destroyed 75% of this mycotoxin. Also, the use of ammonium carbonate at a temperature of 132°C has destroyed 92% [28]. Therefore, with increasing temperature, we will see more destruction of this mycotoxin [36].

2.13 Biological methods

In recent years, biological detoxification has received much attention and has become the main trend in the research of detoxification of fungal toxins. Biological detoxification methods mainly include mycotoxin absorption on the microbial cell wall, mycotoxin destruction by microbial metabolites, and the use of effective plant compounds and enzymes [37].

Microorganisms that are used to detoxify mycotoxins must have characteristics such as the ability to destroy fungal toxins, not interfere with food components, be safe and non-pathogenic, not produce stable metabolites, not changing the smell and the taste and taste of feed, and the need for minimum cost for production [38].

2.13.1 Bacteria

Mycotoxin-degrading bacteria can also be isolated from the rumen, intestinal microbes, water and soil. *Flavobacterium aurantiacum* was the first microorganism used for mycotoxin removal. This bacterium metabolizes aflatoxin and converts it into products that are soluble in water, chloroform, and CO_2 [39].

Also, bacteria such as *Bacillus, Pseudomonas*, yeast and fungi belonging to the genus *Trichoderma* are the most important biological control agents against plant pathogens and the production of mycotoxins [40].

The most extensive studies on mycotoxin-degrading microorganisms are related to the microorganism *Eubacterium* BBSH 797, which was isolated from cow rumen fluid. This bacterium has a diepoxidasetolide enzyme that is effective in reducing the toxicity of mycotoxins. *Eubacterium* BBSH 797 is the only microorganism that is used commercially [39].

Other types of bacteria that break down mycotoxins in laboratory conditions (none of them have been tested *in vivo*) include *Flavobacterium aurantiacum*, *Rhodococcuserythropolis*, *Mycobacterium fluoranthenivorans*, *Nocardia asteroids, Corynebacterium rubrum* and *Pseudomonas fluorescens.*

Some lactic acid bacteria can also remove mycotoxins from the culture medium. For example, *Lactobacillus rhamnosus* GG (LGG) strain is the most effective bacteria for removing aflatoxin and zearalenone from the liquid culture medium [41].

In a study using five probiotic bacteria *Lactobacillus acidophilus, Lactobacillus reuteri, Bifidobacterium bifidum, Lactobacillus johnsonii, Lactobacillus rhamnosus,* it was shown that they can bind and remove mutagenic toxins such as aflatoxin M1 [39].

In a report, it has been shown that some *Pseudomonas species* such as *P. putida, Pseudomonas aeruginosa* can remove AFB1 by 90% during 24-hour incubation. In another study, mycotoxin degradation by 32 species of *Rhodococcus* strain has been investigated. The results showed that 59% of *Rhodococcus* strains decompose more than 90% of AFB1 and remove its genotoxicity [42].

Enterococcus faecium is another bacterium that detoxifies this mycotoxin by attaching AFB1 to its cell wall under the influence of peptidoglycan and polysaccharides [43]. Based on the studies, there is a synergistic effect between the strains of bacteria that play a role in the detoxification of mycotoxins. For example, the use of a group of mycotoxin-decomposing bacteria in a study caused the simultaneous destruction of AFB1 and Ziralenone [28].

2.13.2 Detoxification activity of lactic acid bacteria (LAB)

Lactic acid bacteria (LAB) have various applications in the food industry and are among the effective bacteria in reducing the toxicity of mycotoxins. LAB is superior to other microorganisms in reducing mycotoxins for the following reasons: they are naturally present in the intestines and they have a high biodiversity and are easily cultivated. But the use of LAB also has disadvantages, such as changing the smell and taste of food, the possibility of changing the nutritional value, and slight reversibility in binding to poison [44]. In **Table 1**, the applications of lactic acid to destroy fungal toxins are mentioned.

	Reference	Microorganism	Target Mycotoxin	Degradation%
1.	[45]	*Lactobacillus rhamnosus GG, L. rhamnosus*	Aflatoxin B1	80%
2.	[46]	*L. amylovorus, L. rhamnosus*	Aflatoxin B1	50%
3.	[47]	*L. casei, Lactobacillus brevis, Lactobacillus plantarum*	Aflatoxines (B1, B2, G1, G2)	50%
4.	[48]	*L. casei*	Aflatoxin B1	49.2%
5.	[49]	*L. paracase, L. brevis, L. plantarum*	Aflatoxin B1	39–55%
6.	[50]	Lactic acid bacteria strains	Aflatoxins B1 and B2	ND
7.	[47]	*L. casei, L. brevis, L. plantarum*	Ochratoxin A	50%
8.	[51]	*L. acidophilus, Bifidobacterium animalis*	Patulin Ochratoxin A	95% 80%
9.	[52]	*Pediococcus parvulus*	Ochratoxin A	90%
10.	[53]	*L. rhamnosus C*	Ochratoxin A	97%
11.	[54]	*L. brevis 20,023*	Patulin	ND
12.	[55]	*L. plantarum*	Deoxynivalenol	56–66%
13.	[56]	Lactic acid bacteria strains	Deoxynivalenol, tumonisins B1, tumonisins B2	55% 82% 100%
14.	[57]	*L. rhamnosus, L. plantarum A1*	Zearalenone	ND
15.	[58]	*L. paracasei, Lactococcus lactis*	Zearalenone	55%

Table 1.
Applications of lactic acid to destroy fungal toxins in food.

2.13.2.1 Mechanisms of mycotoxin degradation by lactobacillus

Although the mechanism of mycotoxin degradation has not been properly determined, some studies have defined mechanisms for it:

2.13.2.2 Production of active metabolites

Carbon dioxide, phenyllactic acid and hydrogen peroxide bind to mycotoxin and reduce toxicity. Types of proteolytic enzymes, including protease, are produced. Proteolytic enzymes play the most important role in the detoxification properties of LAB. Due to the presence of peptidoglycan, polysaccharides and proteins [44].

Bacteria for the production of probiotic products are selected which are very good for reducing aflatoxins in food, especially milk [59].

2.14 Detoxification activity of yeasts

Yeasts are also effective in breaking down and absorbing mycotoxins. They can play a role by directly affecting mycotoxin synthesis or removing toxins from agricultural products. Among the advantages of yeasts are low nutritional requirements and high resistance to growth on dry surfaces and they are not allergenic like mushrooms [60].

In a study, *Saccharomyces cerevisiae* yeast has significantly reduced DON toxicity. It has also reduced the effects of ochratoxin A and AFB1 in chicken feed [61]. Yeasts remove patulin in fermented foods through physical absorption. And in another study, Yarrow lipolytica yeast has eliminated 50% of ochratoxin concentration [62].

Yeasts remove patulin from fermented foods through physical absorption. In another study, *Yarrowlipolytica* yeast has eliminated 50% of ochratoxin concentration. Also, *Rhodotorula* yeast mucilaginosa has reduced patulin toxin by 50% [63].

Studies have shown that the absorption of mycotoxins by yeasts is the functional carbohydrates present in their cell walls [64]. *Trichosporon mycotoxinivoran* is a yeast that has been isolated from the posterior intestine of termites and is used commercially to remove mycotoxins. This yeast neutralizes OTN and ZON and turns them into non-toxic metabolites [65].

2.15 Detoxification activity of molds

It is interesting to know that molds that can produce mycotoxins are usually able to destroy mycotoxins due to the use of toxin degradation products. For example, non-toxic species of *Aspergillus parasiticus* and *Aspergillus flavus* in corn, peanuts and pistachios have caused the removal of aflatoxin [66].

The use of non-toxic molds in the soil around agricultural products leads to competition with toxic molds and protection against plants infected with toxic molds. They also increase the shelf life of products [67]. In a study, *Trichoderma rici* and *Rhizopus oryza* have reduced aflatoxins AFM1, AFG2, AFG1, AFB1, and AFB2. Also, *Rhizopus, Trichoderma*, and *Penicillium* molds have been used for the biological control of mycotoxins [68]. *Fusarium verticilioidis* is a non-toxic species of *Fusarium*, it has neutralized the toxic species of *Fusarium*, but unfortunately, it is a plant pathogen [69].

2.16 Detoxification activity of enzymes

Now, biotechnology has taken many steps to neutralize mycotoxins with enzymes, which are harmless and environmentally friendly. Enzymes cause detoxification through pathways such as hydrogenation, decarboxylation, oxidation, methylation, esterification, demethylation, and deamination. Depending on the nature, Mycotoxins may activate any of these pathways. Studies have reported the effects of enzymes on aflatoxin, fumonaisin and ochratoxin [70].

Doxynivalenone is the most common mycotoxin in agricultural products. Due to its structure and having a polar part, it is difficult for anti-toxin agents to stick to this mycotoxin. But now, by using esterase enzyme, by cutting its lactone ring, which is irreversible, they have been able to cause the decomposition of this mycotoxin [71].

Since several mycotoxins are usually produced in one product at the same time, we have to use several enzymes to break them down or an enzyme that has the ability to affect several toxins. Cytochromes are also capable of breaking down various mycotoxins such as strigmatocystin, aflatoxin and trichocene. However, the effect of many enzymes such as isomerases and lyases on mycotoxins is still unknown [72].

It is worth mentioning that enzymes may affect the composition of food, including fat, or they may be affected by factors such as humidity and acidity. It is also possible that the mycotoxin is under the protection of food components, in which case it requires pre-treatment for a better effect of the enzymes [71].

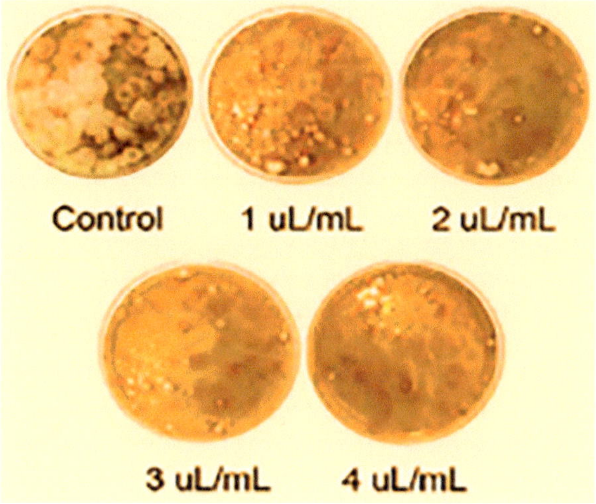

Figure 3.
The inhibitory effect of turmeric essential oil against the growth of Aspergillus flavus *after 5 days of incubation in laboratory conditions [75].*

2.17 Anti-toxic properties of effective plant compounds

The antimicrobial and antioxidant properties of effective plant compounds (essential oils and plant extracts) have been confirmed for years. Now, due to properties such as lipophilicity and low molecular weight, they can easily pass through the cell membrane. They have low toxicity for mammals. Therefore, they have a high potential in the biological control of fungi and mycotoxin production [73].

Many studies have been done in this field, including the study of Ponzilacqua et al., who noticed the destruction of 63.2% of AFB1 by the plant extract *Rosmarinus officinalis* was incubated for 48 hours. Also, some studies have shown the effectiveness of plant extracts on AFB1 in rice and corn [74].

In another study, the detoxification effect of 31 plant extracts against AFB1 was investigated. The results showed that the leaf extract of *Adhatoda vasica* Nees destroys aflatoxin up to 90% at 37 temperature and for 24 hours [15]. The study of Panda and Mehta has shown the destructive effect of 42% of AFB1 by the aqueous extract of *Ocimum tenuiflorum* plant [15].

In a study, the antifungal effect of turmeric essential oil on the mycelium and spores of *Aspergillus flavus* was investigated in different doses in laboratory conditions after 5 days. The results showed significant antifungal activity of the essential oil, which is dependent on the dose [75]. The results of this study can be seen in **Figure 3**.

3. Conclusion

Food contamination with mycotoxins poses serious risks to humans and animals. According to FAO reports, a quarter of agricultural products around the world may be contaminated with mycotoxins. In this study, a review of the methods of detoxification and reduction of mycotoxins in food has been done. Although some specific methods can reduce the level of certain mycotoxins, no single method can be effective against a wide range of mycotoxins that may be present simultaneously in the same product. The effectiveness of physical methods of dealing with mycotoxins is mostly unreliable and is associated with a small yield loss. In addition, many of these physical methods are expensive and can cause a reduction or destruction of the value of the food in it. On the other hand, chemical methods not only require appropriate reaction facilities but also rely on other often time-consuming and expensive operations such as drying and cleaning. Also, only a few chemicals with detoxification capabilities perform detoxification without negatively affecting food value. Among the stated solutions, biological methods are a relatively new approach that has become a safe and reliable solution. Among the other advantages of biological methods that have made them widely used are low cost, minimal impact on food components, easy training, and suitability for all types of solid and liquid foods. However, this method has limitations such as the mechanism of mycotoxin removal with microorganisms and the proper administration of enzymes for optimal enzyme efficiency are being investigated. Therefore, biological methods are effective in removing mycotoxins and are being developed.

Acknowledgements

This study was supported by Tehran University of Medical Sciences.

Conflict of interest

The authors declare that there is no conflict of interest.

Author details

Mehdi Fathollahi[1], Razieh Noroozi[1], Parisa Shavali-gilani[1] and Ebrahim Molaee-aghaee[1,2]*

1 Division of Food Safety and Hygiene, Department of Environmental Health Engineering, School of Public Health, Tehran University of Medical Sciences, Tehran, Iran

2 Department of Food Science and Technology, School of Nutritional Sciences and Dietetics, Tehran University of Medical Sciences, Tehran, Iran

*Address all correspondence to: emolaeeaghaee@tums.ac.ir

References

[1] Magan N, Olsen M. Mycotoxins in Food: Detection and Control. Abington, Cambridge, England: Woodhead Publishing Limited; 2004. Available from: www.woodhead-publishing.com

[2] Agriopoulou S, Stamatelopoulou E, Varzakas T. Advances in occurrence, importance, and mycotoxin control strategies: Prevention and detoxification in foods. Food. 2020;**9**(2):137

[3] Ismaiel AA, Papenbrock J. Mycotoxins: Producing fungi and mechanisms of phytotoxicity. Agriculture. 2015;**5**(3):492-537

[4] Leibetseder J. Decontamination and detoxification of mycotoxins. Biology of Growing Animals. 2006;**4**:439-465

[5] Enyiukwu D, Awurum A, Nwaneri J. Mycotoxins in stored agricultural products: Implications to food safety and health and prospects of plant-derived pesticides as novel approach to their management. Greener Journal of Microbiology and Antimicrobials. 2014;**2**(3):32-48

[6] Yvv A et al. Mycotoxin strategies: Impact on global health and wealth. Pharmaceutica Analytica Acta. 2016;7(7):1-11

[7] Ames I. Mycotoxins, Economic and Health Risks. Ames, IA: CAST (Council of Agricultural Science and Technology), Task force Report; 1989. p. 116

[8] Lutfy O et al. Some control strategies in agricultural grain driers: A review. Journal of Food Agriculture and Environment. 2008;**6**(2):74

[9] Magan N, Evans P. Volatiles as an indicator of fungal activity and differentiation between species, and the potential use of electronic nose technology for early detection of grain spoilage. Journal of Stored Products Research. 2000;**36**(4):319-340

[10] Shi H, Stroshine RL, Ileleji K. Aflatoxin reduction in corn by cleaning and sorting. In: 2014 Montreal, Quebec Canada July 13–July 16, 2014. St. Joseph, Michigan: American Society of Agricultural and Biological Engineers; 2014. Available from: www.asabe.org

[11] Beaver RW. Decontamination of mycotoxin-containing foods and feedstuffs. Trends in Food Science & Technology. 1991;**2**:170-173

[12] Viviane I et al. Mycotoxin's infections and prevention methods: State of the art. Agricultural Sciences. 2021;**12**:1269-1285

[13] Samarajeewa U et al. Detoxification of aflatoxins in foods and feeds by physical and chemical methods. Journal of Food Protection. 1990;**53**(6):489-501

[14] Iqbal SZ et al. Variation of deoxynivalenol levels in corn and its products available in retail markets of Punjab, Pakistan, and estimation of risk assessment. Toxins. 2021;**13**(5):296

[15] Guo Y et al. Novel strategies for degradation of aflatoxins in food and feed: A review. Food Research International. 2021;**140**:109878

[16] Calado T et al. Gamma irradiation effects on ochratoxin A: Degradation, cytotoxicity and application in food. Food Chemistry. 2018;**240**:463-471

[17] Nguyen NX et al. Oil characterization and aflatoxin profile of peanut kernel subjected to gamma-irradiation.

International Journal of Food Engineering. 2020;**6**(1):2-6

[18] Nemțanu MR et al. Inactivation effect of electron beam irradiation on fungal load of naturally contaminated maize seeds. Journal of the Science of Food and Agriculture. 2014;**94**(13):2668-2673

[19] Herzallah S, Alshawabkeh K, Fataftah AA. Aflatoxin decontamination of artificially contaminated feeds by sunlight, γ-radiation, and microwave heating. Journal of Applied Poultry Research. 2008;**17**(4):515-521

[20] Pillai SD, Shayanfar S. Electron beam technology and other irradiation technology applications in the food industry. In: Applications of Radiation Chemistry in the Fields of Industry, Biotechnology and Environment. Cham: Springer; 2017. pp. 249-268

[21] Abuagela MO et al. Assessing pulsed light treatment on the reduction of aflatoxins in peanuts with and without skin. International Journal of Food Science & Technology. 2018;**53**(11):2567-2575

[22] Gavahian M et al. Combinations of emerging technologies with fermentation: Interaction effects for detoxification of mycotoxins? Food Research International. 2021;**141**:110104

[23] Ten Bosch L et al. Plasma-based degradation of mycotoxins produced by *Fusarium*, *Aspergillus* and *Alternaria* species. Toxins. 2017;**9**(3):97

[24] Wu Y, Cheng JH, Sun DW. Blocking and degradation of aflatoxins by cold plasma treatments: Applications and mechanisms. Trends in Food Science & Technology. 2021;**109**:647-661

[25] Kalagatur NK et al. Effect of high pressure processing on growth and mycotoxin production of *Fusarium graminearum* in maize. Food Bioscience. 2018;**21**:53-59

[26] Jouany JP. Methods for preventing, decontaminating and minimizing the toxicity of mycotoxins in feeds. Animal Feed Science and Technology. 2007;**137**(3-4):342-362

[27] Zachetti VG et al. Preliminary study on the use of chitosan as an eco-friendly alternative to control Fusarium growth and mycotoxin production on maize and wheat. Pathogens. 2019;**8**(1):29

[28] Wang Y et al. Simultaneous degradation of aflatoxin B1 and zearalenone by a microbial consortium. Toxicon. 2018;**146**:69-76

[29] Martínez K et al. The effect of edible chitosan coatings incorporated with *Thymus capitatus* essential oil on the shelf-life of strawberry (Fragaria × ananassa) during cold storage. Biomolecules. 2018;**8**(4):155

[30] Yang K et al. Effect of ozone and electron beam irradiation on degradation of zearalenone and ochratoxin A. Toxins. 2020;**12**(2):138

[31] Soares C et al. Use of IoT to real-time monitoring of storage silo and ozone gas fungal decontamination strategy. International Journal of Computers and Applications. 2020;**175**(16):1-7

[32] Wang L et al. Effect of ozone treatment on deoxynivalenol and wheat quality. PLoS One. 2016;**11**(1):e0147613

[33] Luo X et al. Effect of ozone treatment on aflatoxin B1 and safety evaluation of ozonized corn. Food Control. 2014;**37**:171-176

[34] Rastegar H et al. Removal of aflatoxin B1 by roasting with lemon

juice and/or citric acid in contaminated pistachio nuts. Food Control. 2017;**71**:279-284

[35] Kabak B, Dobson AD, Var I. Strategies to prevent mycotoxin contamination of food and animal feed: A review. Critical Reviews in Food Science and Nutrition. 2006;**46**(8):593-619

[36] Borràs-Vallverdú B et al. Deoxynivalenol degradation in wheat kernels by exposition to ammonia vapours: A tentative strategy for detoxification. Food Control. 2020;**118**:107444

[37] Nešić K, Habschied K, Mastanjević K. Possibilities for the biological control of mycotoxins in food and feed. Toxins. 2021;**13**(3):198

[38] Varga J, Tóth B. Novel strategies to control mycotoxins in feeds: A review. Acta Veterinaria Hungarica. 2005;**53**(2):189-203

[39] Çelik K et al. Current developments in removal of mycotoxins by biological methods and chemical adsorbents. Journal of Hygienic Engineering and Design. 2013;**3**:17-20

[40] Afshar P et al. Aflatoxins biodetoxification strategies based on probiotic bacteria. Toxicon. 2020;**178**:50-58

[41] Serrano-Niño J et al. Assessment of probiotic strains ability to reduce the bioaccessibility of aflatoxin M1 in artificially contaminated milk using an *in vitro* digestive model. Food Control. 2013;**31**(1):202-207

[42] Eshelli M et al. Metabolomics of the bio-degradation process of aflatoxin B1 by actinomycetes at an initial pH of 6.0. Toxins. 2015;7(2):439-456

[43] Umesha S et al. Aflatoxins and food pathogens: Impact of biologically active aflatoxins and their control strategies. Journal of the Science of Food and Agriculture. 2017;**97**(6):1698-1707

[44] Wu Q et al. Biological degradation of aflatoxins. Drug Metabolism Reviews. 2009;**41**(1):1-7

[45] El-Nezami H et al. Ability of dairy strains of lactic acid bacteria to bind a common food carcinogen, aflatoxin B1. Food and Chemical Toxicology. 1998;**36**(4):321-326

[46] Peltonen K et al. Aflatoxin B1 binding by dairy strains of lactic acid bacteria and bifidobacteria. Journal of Dairy Science. 2001;**84**(10):2152-2156

[47] Niderkorn V et al. Cell wall component and mycotoxin moieties involved in the binding of fumonisin B1 and B2 by lactic acid bacteria. Journal of Applied Microbiology. 2009;**106**(3):977-985

[48] Hernandez-Mendoza A, Garcia H, Steele J. Screening of *Lactobacillus casei* strains for their ability to bind aflatoxin B1. Food and Chemical Toxicology. 2009;**47**(6):1064-1068

[49] Śliżewska K, Smulikowska S. Detoxification of aflatoxin B1 and change in microflora pattern by pro biotic *in vitro* fermentation of broiler feed. Journal of Animal and Feed Sciences. 2011;**20**(20):300-309

[50] Biernasiak J, Piotrowska M, Libudzisz Z. Detoxification of mycotoxins by probiotic preparation for broiler chickens. Mycotoxin Research. 2006;**22**:230-235

[51] Fuchs S et al. Detoxification of patulin and ochratoxin A, two abundant mycotoxins, by lactic acid bacteria.

Food and Chemical Toxicology. 2008;**46**(4):1398-1407

[52] Abrunhosa L et al. Biodegradation of ochratoxin A by *Pediococcus parvulus* isolated from Douro wines. International Journal of Food Microbiology. 2014;**188**:45-52

[53] Luz C et al. Toxicity reduction of ochratoxin A by lactic acid bacteria. Food and Chemical Toxicology. 2018;**112**:60-66

[54] Wang L et al. A new insight into the adsorption mechanism of patulin by the heat-inactive lactic acid bacteria cells. Food Control. 2015;**50**:104-110

[55] Franco T et al. Lactic acid bacteria in the inhibition of *Fusarium graminearum* and deoxynivalenol detoxification. Journal of Applied Microbiology. 2011;**111**(3):739-748

[56] Niderkorn V, Boudra H, Morgavi D. Binding of *Fusarium* mycotoxins by fermentative bacteria *in vitro*. Journal of Applied Microbiology. 2006;**101**(4):849-856

[57] Čvek D et al. Adhesion of zearalenone to the surface of lactic acid bacteria cells. Hrvatski časopis za prehrambenu tehnologiju, biotehnologiju i nutricionizam. 2012;7(SPECIAL ISSUE-7th):49-52

[58] Rogowska A et al. Investigation of zearalenone adsorption and biotransformation by microorganisms cultured under cellular stress conditions. Toxins. 2019;**11**(8):463

[59] Sanders ME. Lactic acid bacteria as promoters of human health. In: Goldberg I, editor. Functional Foods. Boston, MA: Springer; 1994. DOI: 10.1007/978-1-4615-2073-3_14

[60] El-Tarabily KA, Sivasithamparam K. Potential of yeasts as biocontrol agents of soil-borne fungal plant pathogens and as plant growth promoters. Mycoscience. 2006;**47**:25-35

[61] Mendieta CR et al. Effect of the addition of saccharomyces cerevisiae yeast cell walls to diets with mycotoxins on the performance and immune responses of broilers. The Journal of Poultry Science. 2018;**55**(1):38-46

[62] Yang Q et al. Ochratoxin A is degraded by *Yarrowia lipolytica* and generates non-toxic degradation products. World Mycotoxin Journal. 2016;**9**(2):269-278

[63] Li X et al. Detoxification of mycotoxin patulin by the yeast *Rhodotorula mucilaginosa*. Food Control. 2019;**96**:47-52

[64] Yiannikouris A et al. Alkali extraction of β-D-glucans from *Saccharomyces cerevisiae* cell wall and study of their adsorptive properties toward zearalenone. Journal of Agricultural and Food Chemistry. 2004;**52**(11):3666-3673

[65] Sun X et al. Biological detoxification of zearalenone by *Aspergillus niger* strain FS10. Food and Chemical Toxicology. 2014;**72**:76-82

[66] Horn BW, Dorner JW. Effect of nontoxigenic *Aspergillus flavus* and *A. parasiticus* on aflatoxin contamination of wounded peanut seeds inoculated with agricultural soil containing natural fungal populations. Biocontrol Science and Technology. 2009;**19**(3):249-262

[67] Alberts J et al. Technological and community-based methods to reduce mycotoxin exposure. Food Control. 2017;**73**:101-109

[68] Błaszczyk L et al. Suppressive effect of spp. on toxigenic species. Polish Journal of Microbiology. 2017;**66**(1):85-100

[69] Wagacha J, Muthomi J. Mycotoxin problem in Africa: Current status, implications to food safety and health and possible management strategies. International Journal of Food Microbiology. 2008;**124**(1):1-12

[70] Zhang Z et al. Physical adsorption of patulin by *Saccharomyces cerevisiae* during fermentation. Journal of Food Science and Technology. 2019;**56**:2326-2331

[71] Loi M et al. Mycotoxin biotransformation by native and commercial enzymes: Present and future perspectives. Toxins. 2017;**9**(4):111

[72] Lyagin I, Efremenko E. Enzymes for detoxification of various mycotoxins: Origins and mechanisms of catalytic action. Molecules. 2019;**24**(13):2362

[73] Pawar V, Thaker V. In vitro efficacy of 75 essential oils against *Aspergillus* niger. Mycoses. 2006;**49**(4):316-323

[74] Ponzilacqua B et al. Effects of medicinal herb and Brazilian traditional plant extracts on *in vitro* mycotoxin decontamination. Food Control. 2019;**100**:24-27

[75] Hu Y et al. Mechanisms of antifungal and anti-aflatoxigenic properties of essential oil derived from turmeric (*Curcuma longa* L.) on *Aspergillus flavus*. Food Chemistry. 2017;**220**:1-8

Chapter 5

Research Progress on Prevention and Elimination of Patulin in Food

Xiangfeng Zheng, Zhongyang Cao, Jiang Li and Zhenquan Yang

Abstract

Patulin (PAT) is a highly toxic secondary polyketone metabolite produced by *Penicillium*, *Aspergillus*, *Trichomycosis*, and other fungi, of which *Penicillium expansum* is the main toxigenic strain. Due to its water solubility, acid stability, and heat resistance, PAT often appears in fruits such as apples, peaches, pears, grapes, fruit products (fruit wine, fruit puree, fruit juice, etc.), vegetables, and grains; especially in mildewed apples, PAT residue is very large and difficult to remove. It is necessary to take appropriate methods to prevent and control PAT in products. Although the current common physical, chemical, and biological methods can alleviate the contamination problem of PAT, there are still some limitations, such as insufficient safety assessment of physical and chemical materials and environmental pollution, potential secondary pollution, and insufficient effectiveness of biocontrol and other problems. Therefore, it is necessary to explore the research progress of PAT prevention and detoxification methods and innovative strategies for mycotoxin control. This chapter reviewed the methods and mechanisms used to control the content of PAT in food, and discussed and summarized the possible future trends in the prevention and control of mycotoxins, providing theoretical reference value for solving the problem of PAT contamination in food.

Keywords: PAT, control methods, decontamination, biological control, mechanism

1. Introduction

Patulin (PAT) is one of the major mycotoxins produced by several fungi such as *Aspergillus*, *Trichomycosis*, and *Penicillium* [1], among which *Penicillium expansum* is the main toxigenic fungi. PAT has a variety of toxicity, and its immunotoxicity, reproductive toxicity, dermal toxicity, enterotoxicity, hepatotoxicity, and nephrotoxicity have been found successively, posing a serious threat to human health [2]. According to statistics, the food loss caused by PAT exceeded in developed and developing countries is as high as 25 and 50%, respectively, and the impact of PAT on the development of the food industry has aroused widespread concern in society. Therefore, seeking efficient and economical PAT prevention and control methods has become an important topic of national food industry safety research.

The main methods of mycotoxin removal in food include physical, chemical, and biological methods, which have shown good control effect on PAT in food, and some of them have been used in actual production. The basic principle of PAT elimination is to inhibit the growth of PAT-producing strains and PAT production, or directly remove the accumulated PAT in food. A large amount of literature has reviewed the applicability, mechanisms, advantages, and limitations of different methods [3]. Zheng et al. [3] discussed the regulatory factors of PAT in apple and the regulation of PAT production at the level of protein expression and metabolism, which will promote the development of physical, chemical, and biological methods to control PAT production. Gamal et al. [4] introduced in more detail the possible factors of mycotoxin production and food contamination in the whole food management chain from pre-harvest to post-harvest, which has important reference significance for ensuring that PAT is always at a safe level in the food production process. This study reviewed the basic properties, toxicity, pollution status, prevention, and removal of PAT in order to provide theoretical support for solving the problem of PAT contamination in food.

2. PAT overview

2.1 Basic properties of PAT

PAT is a colorless crystalline water-soluble polyketonolactone with a molecular weight of 154.12 and a melting point of 110.5~112.0°C. It is easily soluble in low pH water and organic solvents such as ethanol, acetone, ethyl acetate, and chloroform, insoluble in petroleum ether but slightly soluble in benzene and ether. PAT has high acid stability even at high temperatures over 100°C, while it is unstable under alkaline conditions [5].

2.2 Toxicity and limit standards of PAT

PAT is toxic to more than 75 species of Gram-positive and Gram-negative bacteria to varying degrees. Initially, PAT was usually used as an antibiotic (**Figure 1**), but later, as it was found that PAT can inhibit fungi and bacteria, and also cause pathogenicity to mammals, including genotoxicity, teratogenicity, carcinogenicity, mutagenicity, etc. (**Figure 2**) [6], so more studies are focusing on PAT as a mycotoxin prevention and control. In view of the broad-spectrum toxicity of the above PAT, a number of countries and institutions have established the maximum limit standard to protect the health of consumers, and the maximum content of PAT in apple juice and apple products is limited to 50 μg/kg, of which the European Union for different production processes and audiences of apple products. More detailed and strict limit standards have been established for PAT content in related products: the maximum PAT content in fruit juice and apple beverages, solid apple products, infant liquid, or solid apple products is 50, 25, and 10 μg/kg, respectively [7]. Despite this, PAT exceedances still occur in some countries, posing a serious threat to human health.

2.3 Present contamination status of PAT

The water solubility of PAT leads to its easy cumulative effect in grains, vegetables, fruits, and their derivatives, especially apples and their derivatives (up

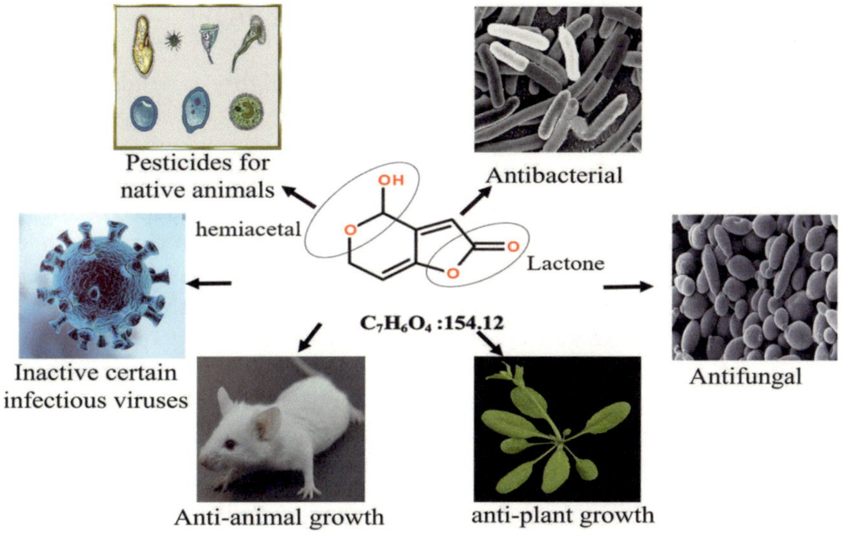

Figure 1.
Chemical structure and biological activities of patulin.

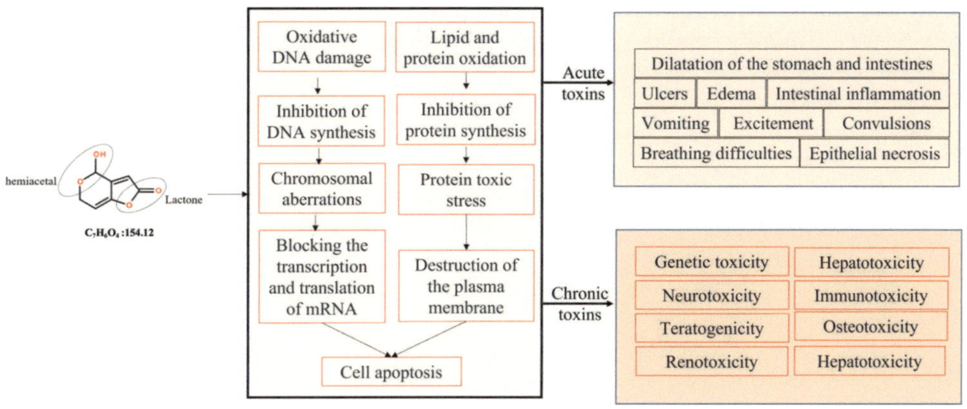

Figure 2.
Toxicity and mode of action of patulin on biological systems.

to 17.5 mg/kg). It has been reported that PAT in human body is mainly ingested through apples and apple products [8]. At the same time, the high temperature resistance of PAT makes it difficult to remove by traditional hot processing or home cooking, so it is easy to cause residue and pollution of PAT in food or feed. Mahato et al. [8] summarized the occurrence of PAT in the world. Among them, developed countries such as the United States, Canada, Portugal, and Belgium and developing countries such as South Africa, Argentina, and Turkey all have a large amount of PAT pollution in fruits and their products. In particular, countries such as Argentina, South Africa, Spain, and Portugal have also detected PAT in baby food. These facts indicate that PAT pollution has posed a major challenge to economic development and public health.

3. The prevention and detoxification methods of PAT

Studies have found that the accumulation of PAT is highly dependent on the strain and has little relationship with different storage steps during the long-term storage of apples [9], so the prevention and control of PAT in food is largely the prevention and control of the toxigenic strains of PAT. Therefore, pre-harvest control (selection of resistant varieties, pest management), harvest control (timely harvesting, manual picking), and post-harvest control (high-pressure washing, cold chain storage) can be selected to prevent the contamination of virus-producing strains of PAT as much as possible [2]. However, contamination can occur at any stage of the food management chain, and it is impossible to guarantee the existence of PAT virus-producing strains and PAT zero in the food chain, so the inhibition of PAT producing strains existing in the contaminated food matrix and the removal of PAT are crucial. Therefore, this review will mainly discuss the prevention and control methods of PAT in food from six aspects: physical, chemical, and biological methods to inhibit virus-producing strains of PAT and to eliminate PAT.

3.1 The growth of PAT-producing strains was inhibited by physical methods

Controlling the growth of PAT-producing fungi is important to reduce the production of PAT, especially for foods that are susceptible to contamination by PAT-producing bacteria during storage, such as apples and their derivatives (**Figure 3**). However, PAT mainly infects apples with *Penicillium* extension of toxigenic bacteria

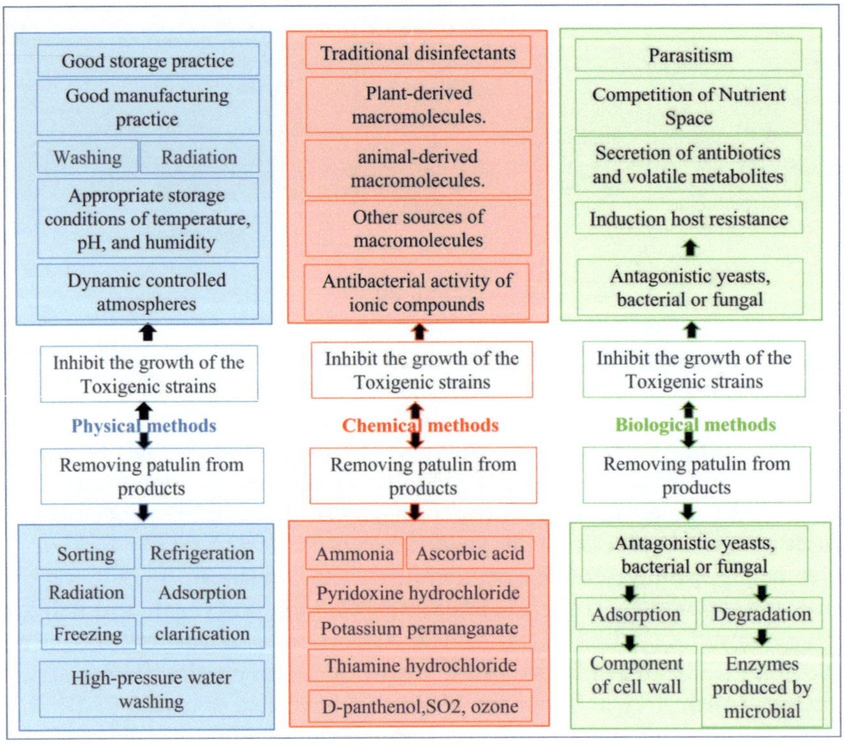

Figure 3.
The prevention and detoxification methods of PAT.

mainly through the wound, so following good manufacturing practice (GMP) and good storage practice (DSP) can effectively ensure the integrity of the surface of the melon and fruit, thereby avoiding the spread of *Penicillium* contamination of apples and their derivatives. Mild hot water treatment can reduce postharvest decay of kiwifruit and enhance the defensive response to *P. expansum* [10]. Appropriate storage environment temperature, pH, and humidity also have significant effects on inhibiting the growth of *Penicillium* extensor and PAT metabolism [11]. DOS et al. [12] evaluated "Fuji Mishima" apples (up to 25% rot) with a respiratory quotient (RQ) of 1.3 on dynamic controlled atmospheres (DCA) and fungal and PAT contamination under different CO_2 partial pressure conditions, and the results showed that PAT accumulation under DCA-RQ storage conditions of 1.3 and 0.8 kPa CO_2 was lower than the maximum allowable level in Brazil. Irradiation method has always been a hot research method because of its easy operation and economic applicability [13, 14]. ZHU et al. [15] recently reported that blue LED light-reduced fungal and mycotoxin pollution by down-regulating the expression of pathogenicity-related genes and PAT biosynthesis-related genes of *P. dilatum*. However, blue LED light treatment (< 0.12 μmol m^{-2} s^{-1}) had a certain impact on apple quality. Chong et al. [16] found that with the aid of food-grade photosensitizer chlorophyll, 405 nm blue LED light inactivated (52.1 ± 7.3)% of *P. expansum* within 30 min on the medium, indicating that chlorophylli-based photosensitization can be used as a method to reduce the risk of *P. expansum* infection. De et al. [17] proved that shortwave ultraviolet (Ultraviolet C) at 277.0-nm and 253.7-nm wavelengths (ultraviolet C). The effect of UV-C (500 mJ/cm^2) on the inactivation of extended penicillium spores on apple peel is equivalent to the washing effect achieved by the industrial use of hypochlorite solution (200 mg/L free chlorine), but this method is only suitable for treating undamaged apples. Therefore, the use of physical methods to control the infection of PAT toxigenic fungal is affected by many factors. At present, cold storage is a common physical method to reduce the contamination of PAT. COTON et al. [18] suggest that apples should be stored in a low temperature environment below 8°C, because the low temperature environment between 8°C and 20°C has little effect on the inhibition of PAT. In addition, even low temperature conditions of 1°C did not prevent the large accumulation of PAT caused by high spore coverage, highlighting the importance of environmental hygiene practices for post-harvest storage. The results above indicate that physical inhibition of virus-producing strains of PAT has its limitations.

3.2 Physical method to remove PAT from the product

A large number of studies have focused on the direct removal of PAT from fruit products by physical methods (**Figure 3**). Studies have shown that physical methods such as picking, high pressure washing, freezing, juice clarification, adsorption, pasteurization, and radiation treatment are effective for removing PAT from products. However, such as picking method, high pressure washing, and other simple methods have a strong selectivity for the type of product, and time consuming, usually used for large and not easy to break apple, citrus, kiwi, and other fruit raw materials. Catana et al. [19] found that PAT content decreased significantly in the process of processing contaminated apple fruit puree, and the thermal stability of PAT in the fruit puree decreased, indicating that it is possible to reduce PAT content in products through food processing. As a method to remove PAT from apple products, adsorption has been widely studied because of its simplicity, economy, and environmental protection. According to research, silica gel, chitosan resin, and other macromolecular porous substances have adsorption effect on PAT in contaminated apple juice and other liquid products. The novel magnetic multi-wall carbon nanotubes synthesized by Zhang et al. [20] have an adsorption efficiency of 0.64 $\mu g\ mg^{-1}/h^{-1}$ for PAT in aqueous solution system, which significantly improves the adsorption efficiency and can separate waste materials through magnetic separation, although magnetic separation technology has not been widely used in the food industry at present. Some other methods, such as water-insoluble corn flour, have been restricted due to economic violations, possible secondary pollution, and inadequate quality assessment [21]. PAT removal methods based on light irradiation have been studied since the 1980s. Ultraviolet irradiation (254 nm, 3.8 mW/cm^2) for 15 min can significantly reduce the toxicity of PAT in apple juice, but this process has a great impact on the color value and ascorbic acid content of apple juice [22]. Moreover, it was found that tannic acid and pigment groups in food substrate had certain influence on the effect of UV light on PAT removal. Funes et al. [23] used pulsed light at doses of 2.4 to 35.8 J/cm^2 to significantly reduce PAT levels in samples. Further analysis by Li et al. [24] showed that the mechanism of PAT degradation by pulsed light was to destroy the lactone ring of PAT to produce DPA with lower toxicity and to maintain the quality of apple juice on the whole.

3.3 The growth of PAT-producing strains was inhibited by chemical methods

Chemical methods show great potential in the prevention and control of PAT pollution (**Figure 3**). Typical traditional fungicides, such as fluroxil, thiazinam, benazim, pyrimethanil, and imazole, have been widely used to prevent the infection of PAT-producing strains in pre-harvest apples. However, in recent years, due to social pressure and strict legislative policies, the search for environmentally friendly alternatives to synthetic chemical-based postharvest treatment methods has become increasingly popular. A number of ionic compounds with antimicrobial activity have been reported. ZHANG et al. [25, 26] studied that ClO_2 fumigation treatment (200 mg/L) can reduce PAT production of *P. expansum* in apple and PDB by 64.83%, and the main mechanism is that the integrity of spore plasma membrane is reduced and cell leakage is caused. Abdalsada et al. [27] found that ZnO had complete inhibition on two PAT virulence bacteria, *P. domatium* and *P. expansum*, at a mass concentration of 5 mg/mL, and the fungi in PDA medium containing ZnO still had strong growth ability in the new medium, indicating that ZnO was not a fungicide. Janczak et al. [28] determined that the bactericidal biocides containing Ag, Cu, ZnO, and $FeCl_3$ were resistant to *Penicillium* expansions. Other chemical agents such as sodium hypochlorite and hydrogen peroxide, boric acid, and potassium phosphate also have good antifungal effects, but the chlorination, oxidation, and hydrolysis of the chemical agents themselves pose a public health challenge. The activity of many macromolecules of plant, animal, or other sources against PAT-producing fungi has been widely discussed. Buonsenso et al. [29] used six essential oils of basil, oregano, mint, thyme, lemon, and fennel vapor to evaluate the control effect on apple blue mildew caused by *P. expansum*, and the results showed that essential oils of basil, oregano, mint, and thyme could effectively inhibit the growth of *P. expansum* silk *in vitro*. Lemon and oregano essential oils have the best effect on reducing blue mold in apple, which may be related to the antibacterial mechanism of different essential oils. The high antimicrobial and antioxidant properties of herbal essential oils explain the efficacy of biofumigation based on plant-derived macromolecules in the control of fungal and mycotoxin contamination after harvest, which would be a possible alternative to fumigants of chemical synthetic substances. The coating of naturally derived edible hydroxypropyl methyl cellulose on apples can reduce postharvest losses associated with *Penicillium* elongate growth and physiological disorders, while maintaining apple hardness and color [30]. Kadium et al. [31] all phenolic compounds extracted from oak and bitter melon showed antibacterial activity against *P. expansum*, among which the phenolic extract of bitter melon had stronger activity, and the antibacterial effect was mainly restricted by concentration. Dou et al. [32] revealed the inhibitory mechanism of ε-polylysine on *P. expansum in vitro* and in apple through transcriptome analysis, which mainly involved damaging the mitochondrial function and membrane integrity of *P. expansum*. Ma et al. [33] found that a monoterpenoid substance could effectively inhibit the mycelial growth of *P. expansum*, but it had an obvious dose-dependent effect on the virulence control of fruit harvesting. Some other reported macromolecules also have such defects when resisting infection by PAT-producing strains, such as flavonoids and total phenols, oligosaccharides [34], tea tree oil [35], cinnamaldehyde and citral combination [36, 37], essential oil caprinaldehyde [38], quercetin [39], jasmonates [40], etc. Considering the conflict between dose cost and antibacterial effect of most plant-derived macromolecules, it is necessary to further explore new, friendly, and economical plant-derived macromolecule products.

3.4 Chemical methods to remove PAT from the product

Currently, chemically cleared PAT is suitable for industrial applications of fruit products (**Figure 3**). A large number of studies have shown that ammonia, ascorbic acid, potassium permanganate, D-calcium pantothenate, thiamine hydrochloride, pyridoxine hydrochloride, SO_2, and ozone can effectively remove PAT in aqueous solution or apple juice. Among them, ammonia and potassium permanganate will produce mutagenic residues, while ascorbic acid, D-calcium pantothenate, thiamine hydrochloride, and pyridoxine hydrochloride have low efficiency for the removal of PAT, so these single methods have been gradually abandoned. Ozone is often used as an oxidizer and disinfectant in food processing and water treatment. Studies have shown that ozone can inactivate toxin-producing fungi and destroy the double bond structure of toxins [41], and has little impact on the quality of processed fruits, vegetables, and juice, so ozone is now mostly used for storing fruits and vegetables and their products. Recently, a class of mercaptan compounds has been shown to be able to purify fruit juices contaminated with PAT. Diao et al. [42] summarized relevant studies on the removal or degradation of PAT by mercaptan compounds in the past few years. As early as 2000, Fliege et al. [43] reported the non-enzymatic reaction mechanism of glutathione (GSH) and N-acetyl-L-cysteine (N-acetyl-L-Cysteine) with PAT in the electrophilic study of PAT. Zhong et al. [44] showed that the mediated binding of cellular antioxidants GSH and PAT played an important role in the degradation of PAT by *Saccharomyces cerevisiae*. Therefore, the increasing interest of researchers in obtaining -SH-containing materials through physical or chemical modification may indicate that the sulfhydryl functionalization of materials is one of the trends in adsorption or degradation of PAT in contaminated fruit juices.

3.5 Biological methods to inhibit the growth of PAT-producing strains

Biological method refers to the use of microbial antagonists to inhibit the growth of pathogenic fungi or microbial fermentation and enzymatic hydrolysis to directly eliminate PAT (**Figure 3**). Some biological antagonists are comparable to chemical fungicides. Biological control method has been paid more and more attention by researchers for its advantages of environmental protection, high efficiency, and low cost, and has gradually developed into a new method to prevent PAT pollution. Antagonistic microorganisms control fruit fungal diseases mainly through fungal parasitism, competition for nutrients and space, secretion of antifungal antibiotics and volatile metabolites, and induction of host resistance. SONG et al. [45] screened a *Bacillus* to combat the yellow crown pear disease caused by *P. expansum* by releasing volatile organic compounds. The organic matter (0.04 μL/mL) could completely inhibit the yellow crown pear penicillium disease after being treated for 48 h, showing great potential of the *P. expansum* control. Bartholomew et al. [46] isolated two non-pathogenic strains of *Aspergillus flavus* 404 and 413, both of which could be used as biological control agents of *Penicillium* in apple. *In vitro* growth activity showed that competitive niche colonization was the main mode of action for reducing rot. Zheng et al. [47] significantly reduced the incidence rate and PAT content of apple caused by *P. expansum* by using the XZ1 obtained from preliminary screening, mainly through three potential mechanisms of competition with *P. expansum* for space and nutrients, secretion of antifungal components, activation of parasitism, and plant hormone signal transduction. In addition, studies have shown that the regulation of extracellular acidification driven by *P. expansum* by yeast can also affect PAT synthesis [48]. Alimadadi et al. [49] selected a total of 50 strains of yeast with antagonistic activity against *P. expansum* by double culture method, among which *Cryptococcus* and *Rudotorulla* had significant inhibitory effect on fungal growth. In addition, *Lactobacillus rhamnosus* (from the Pasteur Institute) [50], *Bacillus mohaiweis* YL-RY0310 [51], *Bacillus cereus* B8W8 [52], *Bacillus anomalis* Wickham [53], *Pichia giyemonda* LMA-Cp01 [54], and other microorganisms have also been reported to have *P. expansum* antagonistic properties. The mechanisms of some of these microbes have not yet been revealed.

3.6 Biological methods for removal of PAT from products

Antagonistic microorganisms that inhibit the growth of PAT-producing fungi may not be able to remove the PAT that has accumulated in the product (**Figure 3**). Therefore, it is necessary to screen the antagonistic microorganisms that can directly remove the existing PAT in food. Up to now, a large number of studies have proved that some bacterial and fungal microorganisms have the potential to become new prevention and control agents for PAT [55].

The removal effect of microorganisms on PAT is mainly through adsorption and degradation. Biodegradation, including microbial fermentation and enzymatic hydrolysis, is an important pathway for many antagonistic microorganisms to remove PAT, and its degradation mechanism has been widely studied. Li et al. [56] proved that *C. hannaensis* completely degraded PAT within 30 h through intracellular enzymes. PAT degradation rates by intracellular and extracellular metabolites of *Bacillus mohaiweis* YL-RY0310 [51] were 62.6 and 56.9%, respectively. After proving the conclusion that yeast degraded PAT through aldo-keto reductase (MgAKR) in the third season in the study by ZHANG et al. [57], further studies found that recombinant expression of MgAKR could use NADPH as a coenzyme to convert PAT into ascladiol *in vitro*, and Lys242 and Leu240 were its main active sites. In addition, MgAKR (0.3 μg/mL) can reduce the PAT in fresh pear juice to 12% without affecting the quality of pear juice. This study has valuable reference value for the development of PAT degrading enzymes. In addition, the whey phosphoribosyl transferase from *Rhodotorula mucilaginossia* has also contributed to the development of PAT degrading enzyme preparations for the food industry. Other microorganisms have also shown high PAT degradation capacity, such as *Aspergillus niger* FS10 [58] (intracellular enzyme), caladium TUS-MM1 [59] (cellular and extracellular metabolites), and *Lactobacillus casei* YZU01 [60] (extracellular enzyme), all of which can degrade by intracellular or extracellular metabolites. Bio-adsorption is another important mechanism for biological control of PAT. Zhang et al. [61] studied the removal effect of CCTCC 93161 on PAT in apple juice at 30°C, which reached 85.88%, and further studied the physical adsorption mechanism of yeast on PAT during aqueous fermentation. The results showed that the interaction of polysaccharides and proteins on yeast cell wall with PAT was the main cause of physical adsorption. El et al. [62] found that the reduction rate of PAT (10 μg/mL) in MRS Medium by *Lactobacillus plantarum* 4F was as high as 88.18%, and C═O, C–H, and N–H were the main functional groups for the adsorption of PAT. Simoes et al. [63] isolated 14 LAB strains from edible olives in Brazil, and the adsorption capacity of PAT was only 23~24%. Other probiotics include *Lactobacillus rhamnosus* 6224 [64], *Lactobacillus acidophilus* ATCC 4356 [65] and *Lactobacillus plantarum* ATCC 8014 [66], *Bacillus subtilis* CICC 10034, CGMCC 1.2182, and *Agrobacterium tumefaciens* CGMCC 1.255 and *Bacillus* DSM451 and other bacteria [67, 68] also showed good effect on adsorption and removal of PAT. In general, the efficiency of biodegradation is higher than the adsorption capacity of living or inactivated cells, but the theoretical safety of the adsorption mechanism is better than that of the degradation mechanism.

4. The application trend of innovative strategies for PAT prevention and control was presented

At present, the traditional physicochemical methods are still used for PAT prevention and treatment in the market, and people are increasingly concerned about the unknown toxic products produced in the physicochemical removal process and the adverse effects on product quality. However, most of the efficient and safe biological methods are still unable to meet the requirements for real application in the food industry. With increasing consumer awareness of food safety and demand for advanced methods to control mycotoxin contamination, toxicity, and accompanying diseases, while expecting negligible or even improved impact on product quality, it is clear that a single technical approach alone cannot meet consumer expectations. There is an urgent need for multiple combined approaches and technologies to safely and effectively reduce PAT levels in foods (**Figure 4**). The combined use of multiple physical or chemical methods has been proven to have better PAT removal capabilities and can break the limitations of a single physical and chemical method to a certain extent, such as separation difficulty and potential secondary pollution. Chemical modification crosslinking of physical adsorbent materials is one of the commonly used methods in PAT removal research, and the safety, adsorption capacity, and separation capacity of adsorbent materials are the most important factors to consider. Liang et al. [69] selected stable and easily separated bacterial cellulose gel film material rich in OH active sites for salinization, and the adsorption capacity of PAT in complex apple juice solution remained (498.78 ± 35.94) μg/g, which was 125 times higher than before modification. Liu et al. [70] converted the OH of chitosan resin into –SH to prepare mercaptan-modified chitosan resin in view of the low PAT adsorption capacity of chitosan resin, and the results showed that the modified resin material had significantly enhanced the ability

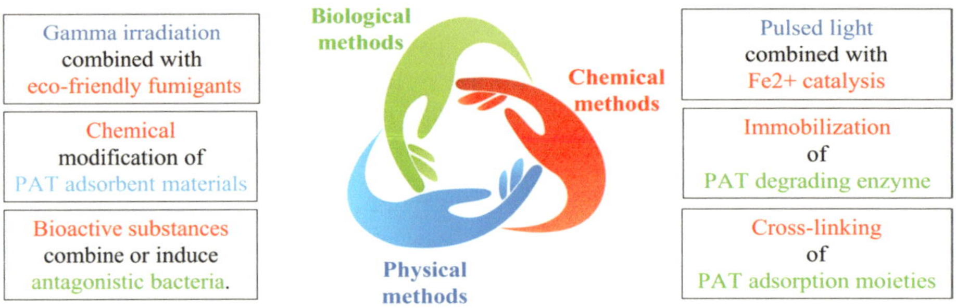

Figure 4.
The trend of innovative strategies for the prevention and control of patulin.

to remove PAT from aqueous solution. Thiourea-polygalacturonic acid complex [71] (polygalacturonic acid plays a major role), cross-linked xanthogenated chitosan resin [72], chlorogenic acid and lignin cross-linked particles [73], and calcium alginate activated carbon beads [74] also showed the same effect. In addition, synergies between physical and chemical methods have been reported in several studies. Rodriguez-Bencomo et al. [75] reported that the ability of exogenous GSH to degrade PAT in apple juice was enhanced by inducing the formation of PAT-GSH conjugates under pulsed light activation or Fe^{2+} catalytic activation. Despite the remarkable results in the degradation effect of PAT, the instability of juice quality after treatment and the high value of GSH limit its application in apple products. Cheon et al. [76] further studied the effect of combined treatment on controlling postharvest rot of stored apples after verifying the *in vitro* anti-*Penicillium* effect of gamma irradiation and environmental protection fumigant acetonitronitrile, and found that combined treatment could reduce the necessary radiation dose to achieve the same inhibitory effect on *P. expansum*. However, this method requires special equipment and cannot be widely used to prevent and control diseases caused by pathogens in postharvest apple. Therefore, the combined use of physical technology and chemical method can improve the shortcomings of the original method to a certain extent, and has practical application potential. The new development of biotechnology methods is mainly to improve the biocontrol effectiveness of antagonistic microorganisms, or to increase the possibility of practical application in purifying contaminated fruits and derived products by strengthening the protection and isolation of biodegradable materials such as inactivated cells and degrading enzymes, and realizing the rapid separation and recycling of biological materials. The fixation of a variety of biomolecules with PAT removal capabilities on the surface of special materials to achieve safe and effective PAT removal has proved to be a promising approach. Yan et al. [77] infiltrated porcine pancreatic lipase into the MOF shell, and the thermal stability was four times higher than that of free porcine pancreatic lipase. The degradation rates of PAT in neutral water, acidic water, and apple juice reached 99.6, 60.9, and 52.6%, respectively. This immobilized enzyme technology also has good storage stability, reusability, and biocompatibility. Yan et al. [78] further used ectopic method and self-assembly strategy to prepare layered mesopore zirconium metal-organic framework aerogel modified by cysteine and porcine pancreatic lipase for continuous flow removal of PAT in apple juice. The device showed high adsorption capacity (38.41 μg/mg) and excellent degradation ability (28.68 μg/mg at 10 μg/mL PAT), and more importantly, it had no significant effect on the quality of apple juice. This study provides a potential scheme for the practical application of continuous flow removal of PAT from apple juice. In addition, Qiu et al. [79] prepared a nano-Fe_3O_4 functionalized inactivated yeast bioadsorbent with a maximum adsorption capacity of 2.69 mg/g for PAT, which basically did not affect the quality of fruit juice. Ge et al. [80] fixed the inactivated prion-producing Candida CICC 1769 on magnetic Fe_3O_4@CTS nanoparticles, which could reduce PAT in citrus juice by more than 90%. Xing et al. [81] fixed short-chain dehydrogenase/reductase on DA/PEI-modified magnetic Fe_3O_4 particles, and the detoxification rate of PAT reached 79.5%. Liu et al. [82] used UiO-66(NH2)@Au as a biomolecular immobilization carrier to successfully fix Cys and used it for PAT removal from apple juice. The results showed that the maximum PAT adsorption capacity of the adsorbent based on the metal-organic framework was 10 times than that of the microbial based bioadsorbent. Liu et al. [83] successfully removed PAT in apple juice by CMC/PEI aerogel doped with GO-SH. Qiu et al. [84] coated mercaptan (–SH) functionalized yeast in AGAR aerogel with the optimal glutaraldehyde crosslinking method, which eliminated the presence of PAT in apple juice and had little effect on its quality. In addition, it is also an important measure to improve the biocontrol effectiveness of antagonistic microorganisms by the induction treatment of elicitor. After the induction of methyl jasmonate, the inhibition effect of *Meyerozyma guilliermondii* on *P. expansum* was enhanced, which effectively reduced the rot of apple penicillium and mycotoxin contamination. To sum up, the superiority of the combination of physicochemical technology and biological method provides a new idea for the development of new PAT cleaning technology.

5. Conclusion

At present, PAT pollution in the diet is still relatively serious, and only relying on good production practices and good quality principles to completely degrade the problem of PAT-contaminated food is unrealistic, so researchers have been committed to the development of new, environmentally friendly, low cost, and high safety PAT decontamination agent, in order to replace the traditional chemical fungicides widely used in the market. This paper summarizes some new materials and new methods with good PAT control effect. Although there are still some limitations, the research proves that these new advances in PAT control and detoxification have improved on the original shortcomings, which indicates that the new research has the application potential in the food industry and may become one of the elements of good practice for food production enterprises in the future.

Author details

Xiangfeng Zheng, Zhongyang Cao, Jiang Li and Zhenquan Yang*
Yangzhou University, Yangzhou, China

*Address all correspondence to: 18796002921@163.com

References

[1] Ioi JD, Zhou T, Tsao R, et al. Mitigation of patulin in fresh and processed foods and beverages. Toxins. 2017;**9**(5):157

[2] Barad S, Sionov E, Prusky D. Role of patulin in post-harvest diseases. Fungal Biology Reviews. 2016;**30**(1):24-32

[3] Zheng X, Wei W, Zhou W, et al. Prevention and detoxification of patulin in apple and its products: A review. Food Research International. 2021;**140**:110034

[4] Hamad GM, Mehany T, Simal-Gandara J, et al. A review of recent innovative strategies for controlling mycotoxins in foods. Food Control. 2023;**144**:109350

[5] Moake MM, Padilla-Zakour OI, Worobo RW. Comprehensive review of patulin control methods in foods. Comprehensive Reviews in Food Science and Food Safety. 2005;**4**(1):8-21

[6] Brand B, Stoye NM, Guilherme MDS, et al. Identification of patulin from *Penicillium coronium* as a toxin for enteric neurons. Molecules. 2019;**24**(15):2776

[7] Ji X, Li R, Yang H, et al. Occurrence of patulin in various fruit products and dietary exposure assessment for consumers in China. Food Control. 2017;**78**:100-107

[8] Mahato DK, Kamle M, Sharma B, et al. Patulin in food: A mycotoxin concern for human health and its management strategies. Toxicon. 2021;**198**:12-23

[9] De CN, Vlaemynck G, Van PE, et al. Patulin production by *Penicillium expansum* isolates from apples during different steps of long-term storage. World Mycotoxin Journal. 2016;**9**(3):379-388

[10] Chen HZ, Cheng Z, Wisniewski M. Ecofriendly hot water treatment reduces postharvest decay and elicits defense response in kiwifruit. Environmental Science and Pollution Research. 2015;**22**(19):15037-15045

[11] Tannous J, Atoui A, El KA, et al. A study on the physicochemical parameters for *Penicillium expansum* growth and patulin production: Effect of temperature, pH, and water activity. Food Science & Nutrition. 2016;**4**(4):611-622

[12] Dos SID, Fontana M, Klein B, et al. Fungal growth, patulin accumulation and volatile profile in 'Fuji Mishima' apples under controlled atmosphere and dynamic controlled atmosphere. Food Additives & Contaminants. Part A, Chemistry, Analysis, Control, Exposure & Risk Assessment. 2022;**39**(1):170-184

[13] Adhikari A, Syamaladevi RM, Killinger K, et al. Ultraviolet-C light inactivation of *Escherichia coli* 0157 and listeria monocytogenes on organic fruit surfaces. International Journal of Food Microbiology. 2015;**210**:136-142

[14] Santo D, Graca A, Nunes C, et al. Survival and growth of *Cronobacter sakazakii* on fresh-cut fruit and the effect of UV-C illumination and electrolyzed water in the reduction of its population. International Journal of Food Microbiology. 2016;**231**:10-15

[15] Zhu R, Wang W, Luo Z, et al. Blue LED light treatment inhibits virulence and patulin biosynthesis in *Penicillium expansum*. Postharvest Biology and Technology. 2023;**200**:112340

[16] Chong L, Ghate V, Seah C, et al. Photosensitization can be an effective risk-reduction strategy against the post-baking mold spoilage of bread. Food Microbiology. 2024;**117**:104390-104390

[17] De SVR, Popovic V, Warriner K, et al. A comparative study on the inactivation of *Penicillium expansum* spores on apple using light emitting diodes at 277 nm and a low-pressure mercury lamp at 253.7 nm. Food Control. 2020;**110**:107039

[18] Coton M, Bregier T, Poirier E, et al. Production and migration of patulin in *Penicillium expansum* molded apples during cold and ambient storage. International Journal of Food Microbiology. 2020;**313**:108377

[19] Catana M, Catana L, Iorga E, et al. Assessment of the thermal stability of patulin in apple puree and of possibilities for reduction of patulin contamination level through apple processing. Revista de Chimie. 2018;**69**(4):809-814

[20] Zhang Z, Zeng C, Peng B. Adsorption properties of magnetic carbon nanotubes for patulin removal from aqueous solution systems. Food Control. 2019;**102**:1-10

[21] Guo C, Guo M, Zhang S, et al. Assessment of patulin adsorption efficacy from aqueous solution by water-insoluble corn flour. Journal of Food Safety. 2018;**38**(1):e12397

[22] Diao E, Chu X, Hou H, et al. Improving the safety of apple juice by UV irradiation. Journal of Food Measurement and Characterization. 2018;**12**(3):2005-2011

[23] Funes GJ, Gomez PL, Resnik SL, et al. Application of pulsed light to patulin reduction in McIlvaine buffer and apple products. Food Control. 2013;**30**(2):405-410

[24] Li Y, Cai R, Fu C, et al. Degradation of patulin in apple juice by pulsed light and its effect on the quality. Food and Bioprocess Technology. 2023;**16**(4):870-880

[25] Zhang X, Fu M, Chen Q. Effect of chlorine dioxide (ClO2) on patulin produced by *Penicillum expansum* and involved mechanism. Journal of the Science of Food and Agriculture. 2019;**99**(4):1961-1968

[26] Zhang X, Fu M. Inhibitory effect of chlorine dioxide (ClO2) fumigation on growth and patulin production and its mechanism in *Penicillum expansum*. LWT. 2018;**96**:335-343

[27] Abdalsada MH, Hassan BM. Efficacy of ZnO nanoparticle in inhibiting *Penicillium crustose* and *Penicillium expansum* producers of patulin toxin. Biochemical and Cellular Archives. 2020;**20**(2):3663-3668

[28] Janczak K, Kosmalska D, Kaczor D, et al. Bactericidal and fungistatic properties of LDPE modified with a biocide containing metal nanoparticles. Materials. 2021;**14**(15):4228

[29] Buonsenso F, Schiavon G, Spadaro D. Efficacy and mechanisms of action of essential oils' vapours against blue mould on apples caused by *Penicillium expansum*. International Journal of Molecular Sciences. 2023;**24**(3):2900

[30] Fernandez CP, Gine BJ, Perez GMB, et al. A hydroxypropyl methylcellulose (HPMC)-based coating inhibits ethylene-dependent quality changes and reduces superficial scald incidence and blue mould severity during postharvest handling of two apple varieties. Postharvest Biology and Technology. 2024;**207**:112610

[31] Kadium SW, Abd AASE, Sahib RA. Antifungal activity of phenols compound

separated from quercus infectoria and citrullus colocynthis against toxic fungi. Archives of Razi Institute. 2023;**78**(1):297-303

[32] Dou Y, Dhanasekaran S, Ngea GLN, et al. Transcriptome analysis provides insights into potential mechanisms of epsilon-poly- L-lysine inhibiting *Penicillium expansum* invading apples. Postharvest Biology and Technology. 2024;**207**:112622

[33] Ma D, Ji D, Liu J, et al. Efficacy of methyl thujate in inhibiting *Penicillium expansum* growth and possible mechanism involved. Postharvest Biology and Technology. 2020;**161**:111070

[34] Sui Y, Ma Z, Meng X. Proteomic analysis of the inhibitory effect of oligochitosan on the fungal pathogen, *Botrytis cinerea*. Journal of the Science of Food and Agriculture. 2019;**99**(5):2622-2628

[35] Li Y, Shao X, Xu J, et al. Effects and possible mechanism of tea tree oil against *Botrytis cinerea* and *Penicillium expansum in vitro* and *in vivo* test. Canadian Journal of Microbiology. 2017;**63**(3):219-227

[36] Wang Y, Feng K, Yang H, et al. Antifungal mechanism of cinnamaldehyde and citral combination against *Penicillium expansum* based on FT-IR fingerprint, plasma membrane, oxidative stress and volatile profile. RSC Advances. 2018;**8**(11):5806-5815

[37] Wang Y, Feng K, Yang H, et al. Effect of cinnamaldehyde and citral combination on transcriptional profile, growth, oxidative damage and patulin biosynthesis of *Penicillium expansum*. Frontiers in Microbiology. 2018;**9**:597

[38] Zhou T, Wang X, Ye B, et al. Effects of essential oil decanal on growth and transcriptome of the postharvest fungal pathogen *Penicillium expansum*. Postharvest Biology and Technology. 2018;**145**:203-212

[39] Zhang M, Xu L, Zhang L, et al. Effects of quercetin on postharvest blue mold control in kiwifruit. Scientia Horticulturae. 2018;**228**:18-25

[40] Ahmadi-Afzadi M, Orsel M, Pelletier S, et al. Genome-wide expression analysis suggests a role for jasmonates in the resistance to blue mold in apple. Plant Growth Regulation. 2018;**85**(3):375-387

[41] Diao E, Liu W, Wang Y, et al. Design and application of ozone detoxification equipment for patulin in contaminated apple juice. Transactions of the Chinese Society of Agricultural. 2018;**34**(12):282-287

[42] Diao E, Ma K, Qian S, et al. Removal of patulin by thiol-compounds: A review. Toxicon. 2022;**205**:31-37

[43] Fliege R, Metzler M. Electrophilic properties of patulin.: N-acetylcysteine and glutathione adducts. Chemical Research in Toxicology. 2000;**13**(5):373-381

[44] Zhong L, Carere J, Mats L, et al. Formation of glutathione patulin conjugates associated with yeast fermentation contributes to patulin reduction. Food Control. 2021;**123**:107334

[45] Song C, Zhang Y, Zhao Q, et al. Volatile organic compounds produced by *bacillus aryabhattai* AYG1023 against *Penicillium expansum* causing blue mold on the Huangguan pear. Microbiological Research. 2024;**278**:127531

[46] Bartholomew HP, Luciano-Rosario D, Bradshaw MJ, et al. Avirulent isolates of *Penicillium chrysogenum* to

control the blue mold of apple caused by *Penicillium expansum*. Microorganisms. 2023;**11**(11):2792

[47] Zheng XF, Zheng LL, Xia FP, et al. Biological control of blue mold rot in apple by *Kluyveromyces marxianus* XZ1 and the possible mechanisms of action. Postharvest Biology and Technology. 2023;**196**:112197

[48] Palmieri D, Miccoli C, Notardonato I, et al. Modulation of extracellular *Penicillium expansum* -driven acidification by *Papiliotrema terrestris* affects biosynthesis of patulin and has a possible role in biocontrol activity. Frontiers in Microbiology. 2022;**13**:973670

[49] Alimadadi N, Pourvali Z, Nasr S, et al. Screening of antagonistic yeast strains for postharvest control of *Penicillium expansum* causing blue mold decay in table grape. Fungal Biology. 2023;**127**(3):901-908

[50] Khan-Mohammadi S, Fadaei V, Mirdamadi S. Characterization of yoghurt supplemented with *Lacticaseibacillus rhamnosus* as a bioprotective antifungal culture. Mljekarstvo. 2023;**73**(1):59-72

[51] Ding Y, Liu F, Yang J, et al. Isolation and identification of *Bacillus mojavensis* YL-RY0310 and its biocontrol potential against *Penicillium expansum* and patulin in apples. Biological Control. 2023;**182**:105239

[52] Khadiri M, Boubaker H, Askarne L, et al. *Bacillus cereus* B8W8 an effective bacterial antagonist against major postharvest fungal pathogens of fruit. Postharvest Biology and Technology. 2023;**200**:112315

[53] Zhao QH, Shi Y, Xu CW, et al. Control of postharvest blue and gray mold in kiwifruit by *Wickerhamomyces anomalus* and its mechanism of antifungal activity. Postharvest Biology and Technology. 2023;**201**:112345

[54] Lopez-Cruz R, Segarra G, Torres R, et al. Biocontrol efficacy of *Meyerozyma guilliermondii* LMA-Cp01 against post-harvest pathogens of fruits. Archives of Phytopathology and Plant Protection. 2023;**56**(13):1003-1020

[55] Ben T, Bochraal Q, Yasir MA. Review: Biotechnology of mycotoxins detoxification using microorganisms and enzymes. Toxicon. 2019;**160**:12-22

[56] Ma J, Godana EA, Yang Q, et al. Effect of the antagonistic yeast *Hannaella sinensison* the degradation of patulin. Biological Control. 2023;**178**:105134

[57] Zhang Y, Zhao QH, Ngea GLN, et al. Biodegradation of patulin in fresh pear juice by an aldo-keto reductase from *Meyerozyma guilliermondii*. Food Chemistry. 2024;**436**:137696

[58] Yang Y, Ji J, Wu S, et al. Efficient biodegradation of patulin by *Aspergillus niger* FS10 and metabolic response of degrading strain. Food. 2023;**12**(2):382

[59] Mita M, Sato R, Kakinuma M, et al. Isolation and characterization of filamentous fungi capable of degrading the mycotoxin patulin. Microbiology. 2023;**12**(4):e1373

[60] Zheng X, Wei W, Rao S, et al. Degradation of patulin in fruit juice by a lactic acid bacteria strain *Lactobacillus casei* YZU01. Food Control. 2020;**112**:107147

[61] Zhang Z, Li M, Wu C, et al. Physical adsorption of patulin by *Saccharomyces cerevisiae* during fermentation. Journal of Food Science and Technology. 2019;**56**(4):2326-2331

[62] El-Oirdi S, Lakhlifi T, Kachmar MR, et al. Patulin removal and biopreservation of apple by three lactic acid bacteria strains isolated from foods. Biocontrol Science and Technology. 2023;**33**(12):1139-1155

[63] Simoes L, Fernandes N, Teixeira J, et al. Brazilian table olives: A source of lactic acid bacteria with antimycotoxigenic and antifungal activity. Toxins. 2023;**15**(1):71

[64] Li J, Liu L, Li C, et al. The ability of *Lactobacillus rhamnosus* to bind patulin and its application in apple juice. Acta Alimentaria. 2020;**49**(1):93-102

[65] Zoghi A, Khosravi-Darani K, Sohrabvandi S, et al. Effect of probiotics on patulin removal from synbiotic apple juice. Journal of the Science of Food and Agriculture. 2017;**97**(8):2601-2609

[66] Zoghi A, Khosravi-Darani K, Sohrabvandi S, et al. Patulin removal from synbiotic apple juice using *Lactobacillus plantarum* ATCC 8014. Journal of Applied Microbiology. 2019;**126**(4):1149-1160

[67] Sajid M, Mehmood S, Niu C, et al. Effective adsorption of patulin from apple juice by using non-cytotoxic heat-inactivated cells and spores of alicyclobacillus strains. Toxins. 2018;**10**(9):344

[68] Wang Y, Yuan Y, Liu B, et al. Biocontrol activity and patulin -removal effects of *Bacillus subtilis*, *Rhodobacter sphaeroides* and *Agrobacterium tumefaciens* against *Penicillium expansum*. Journal of Applied Microbiology. 2016;**121**(5):1384-1393

[69] Liang J, He Q, Zhao Y, et al. Synthesis of sulfhydryl modified bacterial cellulose gel membrane and its application in adsorption of patulin from apple juice. LWT. 2022;**158**:113159

[70] Liu B, Peng X, Chen W, et al. Adsorptive removal of patulin from aqueous solution using thiourea modified chitosan resin. International Journal of Biological Macromolecules. 2015;**80**:520-528

[71] Safajoo S, Sadeghi E, Noroozi R, et al. Synthesis of a new thiourea-polygalacturonic acid nanocomplex adsorbent for removing patulin from apple juice simulator and apple juice. Journal of Food Protection. 2022;**17**(3):231-241

[72] Peng X, Liu B, Chen W, et al. Effective biosorption of patulin from apple juice by cross-linked xanthated chitosan resin. Food Control. 2016;**63**:140-146

[73] Sun YH, Shi JJ, Qi JR, et al. *In vitro* and *in vivo* evaluation of chlorogenic acid-encapsulated lignin on patulin adsorption and alleviation of patulin -induced colonic damage. Journal of Agricultural and Food Chemistry. 2023;**71**(29):11217-11227

[74] Yue T, Guo C, Yuan Y, et al. Adsorptive removal of patulin from apple juice using ca-alginate-activated carbon beads. Journal of Food Science. 2013;**78**(10):1629-1635

[75] Jose RJ, Sanchis V, Vinas I, et al. Formation of patulin -glutathione conjugates induced by pulsed light: A tentative strategy for patulin degradation in apple juices. Food Chemistry. 2020;**315**:126283

[76] Cheon W, Kim YS, Balaraju K, et al. Postharvest disease control of Colletotrichum gloeosporioides and *P. expansum* on stored apples by gamma irradiation combined with fumigation. Plant Pathology. 2016;**32**(5):460-468

[77] Yan XH, Chen K, Jia H, et al. Infiltration of porcine pancreatic lipase

into magnetic hierarchical mesoporous UiO-66-NH_2 metal-organic frameworks for efficient detoxification of patulin from apple juice. Food Chemistry. 2024;**431**:137172

[78] Yan X, Dong X, Zhao Q, et al. Continuous flow removal of patulin by cysteine and porcine pancreatic lipase-modified hierarchical mesoporous zirconium metal-organic framework aerogel for apple juice treatment. Chemical Engineering Journal. 2023;**475**:146472

[79] Qiu Y, Guo H, Guo C, et al. One-step preparation of nano-Fe_3O_4 modified inactivated yeast for the adsorption of patulin. Food Control. 2018;**86**:310-318

[80] Ge N, Xu J, Li F, et al. Immobilization of inactivated microbial cells on magnetic Fe_3O_4@CTS nanoparticles for constructing a new biosorbent for removal of patulin in fruit juice. Food Control. 2017;**82**:83-90

[81] Xing M, Chen Y, Dai W, et al. Immobilized short-chain dehydrogenase/reductase on Fe_3O_4 particles acts as a magnetically recoverable biocatalyst component in patulin bio-detoxification system. Journal of Hazardous Materials. 2023;**448**:130986

[82] Liu M, Wang J, Yang Q, et al. Patulin removal from apple juice using a novel cysteine-functionalized metal-organic framework adsorbent. Food Chemistry. 2019;**270**:1-9

[83] Liu M, Wang J, Wang X, et al. Aerogel doped by sulfur-functionalized graphene oxide with convenient separability for efficient patulin removal from apple juice. Food Chemistry. 2021;**338**:127785

[84] Qiu Y, Zhang Y, Wei J, et al. Thiol-functionalized inactivated yeast embedded in agar aerogel for highly efficient adsorption of patulin in apple juice. Journal of Hazardous Materials. 2020;**388**:121802

Chapter 6

Mycotoxicoses in Humans

Girish Patil, Archana Keche and Madhavi Madkey

Abstract

Mycotoxicosis is a term used to describe a series of toxic conditions caused by the ingestion of food contaminated with the toxins of different saprophytic and phytopathogenic fungi and molds. Mycotoxins are secondary metabolites produced naturally by filamentous fungi. They do not have any known metabolic function but are toxic to humans causing harmful consequences. Contamination of foodstuffs like grains, legumes, and nuts may occur in the field during harvest or storage. Humidity and temperature are the two main determinants of mold growth and toxin production. These toxins are produced by fungal species belonging mainly to genus *Aspergillus, Fusarium, Penicillium* etc. The major mycotoxins produced by these fungi are Aflatoxin B1, Ergot alkaloids, Fumonisins, Patulin, Trichothecene, Zearalenone, and Ochratoxin A. Most mycotoxins are nephrotoxic, hepatotoxic, carcinogenic, immunosuppressive, and mutagenic in animal studies, and they pose a serious threat to human health. Among the different mycotoxins, aflatoxin B1 has been reported as the highest carcinogenic mycotoxin. Mycotoxins have the potential to cause outbreaks too. This chapter will focus on the mechanisms involved in the toxicity of important mycotoxins and their harmful effects on human health.

Keywords: *Aspergillus*, *Fusarium*, mycotoxins, aflatoxin, mycotoxicosis, carcinogen

1. Introduction

The toxins produced by fungi are called *mycotoxins*. They are low molecular weight secondary metabolites having no function in fungal metabolism but can be toxic to humans and animals. The five most common mycotoxins found worldwide are *aflatoxins, zearalenone, deoxynivalenol, fumonisins, and ochratoxin A*. These are produced by fungal species of the three important genera—*Aspergillus, Fusarium, and Penicillium. Mycotoxicosis* is defined as a clinical illness of humans or animals due to ingestion of contaminated food by preformed toxins produced by food-borne filamentous fungi. The study of mycotoxins is called *Mycotoxicology* [1].

Mycotoxins represent the major class of naturally produced toxin that readily contaminates the foodstuffs that are consumed regularly by plants and animals [2]. Contamination occurs either directly or indirectly. In a direct way of contamination, a toxigenic fungus directly infects the food, and the toxin is produced in the food. However, indirect contamination occurs via contamination of food ingredients by a toxigenic fungus, and it has been partially eliminated during processing [3]. *The Food and Agriculture Organization (FAO) suggests that mycotoxins are responsible for contaminating at least 25% of the total food produced in the world* [4]. Most mycotoxins are well known to have toxic consequences on human health, which include acute intoxication, nephrotoxicity, hepatotoxicity, carcinogenicity, immunosuppressive effects, mutagenicity, and alteration in reproductive health and development.

This chapter covers the different mechanisms involved in the toxicity of commonly encountered mycotoxins along with their harmful consequences on human health.

2. Historical perspectives and epidemiology

The poisoning due to mycotoxins has been known to humans since ancient times. *Ergot alkaloids are the earliest known mycotoxins*. Gangrenous ergotism was reported in central Europe from the ninth to the fourteenth century, and convulsive ergotism, which involved the nervous system, was witnessed in Europe and the United States from the late sixteenth to nineteenth centuries. This was confused with *witchcraft and led to the conduction of the Salem Witch Trials in 1692 in Massachusetts, USA,* where 24 males and females were convicted [5]. This instance was mentioned in the novel *"Acceptable Risk" by Robin Cook* in 1995. During world war (1938), an anti-Jewish Nazi propaganda book, titled *Der Giftpilz (The Poisonous Mushroom)*, was widely circulated by Adolf Hitler. In the 1930s, thousands of horses were killed in the USSR due to *Stachybotryotoxicosis. Alimentary toxic aleukia (ATA)* was responsible for the deaths of almost 1,00,000 Russians between 1942 and 1948 [1].

Aflatoxins were discovered during the early 1960s in England as a cause of *Turkey-x-disease*, which was responsible for the loss of 1 lakh birds [1]. In November 1974, an outbreak of *curious liver disease occurred in the districts of Gujarat and Rajasthan*. These areas experienced unseasonal rains contaminating the maize crops. More than 400 individuals were affected, and about 100 people died due to this aflatoxin toxicity [6]. In 1975, there was an outbreak of *convulsive ergotism due to intoxication of clavine alkaloids from Claviceps fusiformis*, affecting around 78 persons without any mortality [7]. *In Kenya (1981), an outbreak of acute hepatitis* due to aflatoxins occurred due to consumption of contaminated maize [8]. From June to September 1987, in the *Kashmir valley, there was an outbreak of trichothecenes* due to the consumption of bread made from rain-damaged wheat, and the patient presents self-limiting gastrointestinal symptoms [9]. Another report came from *Malaysia in 1988, where consuming noodles became fatal for 13 children due to acute hepatic encephalopathy* [10]. In 1997, Bhat et al., from *south India, reported an outbreak of fumonisins* due to consumption of contaminated maize and sorghum, affecting 1325 individuals in 27 villages without mortality [11]. Again in 2004, an outbreak of aflatoxicosis occurred in Kenya due to the consumption of maize heavily contaminated with aflatoxin, causing several hundred deaths [12].

3. Medically important mycotoxins causing mycotoxicosis

The following are the frequently encountered toxins causing risk to human health.

1. Aflatoxins

2. Fumonisins

3. Trichothecenes

4. Zearalenone

5. Ochratoxins

6. Cyclopiazonic acid

7. Ergot alkaloids

8. Patulin

The mechanism of action and the harmful consequences produced by medically important mycotoxins are described below (**Table 1**).

Sr. No.	Mycotoxin	Mechanism of toxicity	Clinical disease	*IARC Classification
1.	Aflatoxin	Inhibition of P53 (tumor suppressor gene) and production of reactive oxygen species	Hepatotoxicity, Hepatocellular Carcinoma, Immunosuppression, Aflatoxicosis, Reye's syndrome, effects on reproduction	Group 1
2.	Fumonisins	Inhibition of ceramide synthase enzyme	Esophageal cancer, neural tube defects, nephrotoxic	Group 2B
3.	Trichothecenes	Inhibition of protein synthesis by binding to 60S subunit and inhibiting peptidyl transferase	Digestive tract disorder, reproductive disorder, ATA (Alimentary toxic aleukia) and immunosupression	Group 3
4.	Zearalenone	Imitation of natural estrogen and competition for estrogen receptors	Reproductive disorder	Group 3
5.	Ochratoxin A	Binding to plasma proteins (albumin) and accumulation in target organs	Nephrotoxicity, Balkan endemic nephropathy (BEN) and chronic interstitial nephropathy (CIN), Carcinogenic	Group 2B
6.	Cyclopiazonic acid	Inhibition of ATPase in the intracellular calcium storage site	Kodua poisoning	
7.	Ergot alkaloids	Alpha adrenergic blockage and vasoconstriction	Gangrenous and convulsive ergotism	
8.	Patulin		Neurologic and gastrointestinal disorders	Group 3

**IARC: International Association on Research for Cancer [13].*

Table 1.
The mechanism of action and the harmful consequences produced by medically important mycotoxins.

3.1 Aflatoxins

The word aflatoxin is derived from the first alphabet of *Aspergillus flavus* toxin [1]. Aflatoxins are chemical derivatives of *difuranocoumarin* and are mainly produced by contaminated foodstuffs like maize, rice, and sorghum [14] and also by soybean, pistachio, groundnuts, almonds, walnut, milk, and milk products, meat [15]. *Aspergillus flavus* and *Aspergillus parasiticus* are the main source and, to a lesser extent, *A. nomius, A. bombycis, A. pseudotamari*, and *A. ochraceoroseus* [16]. The main aflatoxins are *B1, B2, G1, and G2*. This nomenclature is based on their blue or green fluorescence under ultraviolet light [17]. Other aflatoxins like P1, Q1, B2A, and G2A are formed due to further metabolism of aflatoxins inside the host. This is known as biotransformation [18].

Aflatoxins are mainly metabolized in the liver by cytochrome P450. During this process, many intracellular reactive oxygen species (ROS) are produced such as superoxide anion, hydroxyl radical, and hydrogen peroxide (H2O2). The toxicity occurs due to increased oxidative stress which damages the cell membranes, proteins, and nucleic acid (DNA and RNA). This leads to impaired cell function, DNA damage, cytolysis, and apoptosis [19]. In addition, they can cause hepatocarcinoma by inhibition of the tumor suppressor gene (p53) (**Figure 1**) [14].

Aflatoxicosis: It is a type of poisoning caused by the consumption of aflatoxins contaminated food. It presents clinically as either acute severe intoxication or chronic sub-symptomatic aflatoxicosis. Acute causes direct liver damage and may be fatal. Chronic form first presents with nonspecific symptoms like anorexia, weakness, fever, jaundice, etc., and subsequently may progress to hepatomegaly, ascites, and portal hypertension [1].

Hepatotoxicity: Aflatoxins, by their mutagenic and carcinogenic properties, are responsible for the development of *hepatocellular carcinoma (HCC)* in humans. They are now designated as a significant risk factor for HCC, along with the blood-borne hepatitis viruses, that is, hepatitis B virus (HBV) and the hepatitis C virus (HCV) [20]. Now, aflatoxin B1 is categorized as a *Group 1 human carcinogen* by the International Agency on Research on Cancer (IARC) [13]. In addition to this, aflatoxin is also the etiological agent for the development of other liver diseases, such as hepatitis, cirrhosis, and hepatomegaly. *Reye's syndrome*, which presents as encephalopathy and fatty degeneration of the liver, is also thought to be caused by aflatoxins. This is endemic in developing countries and mostly affects children [1]. *Indian*

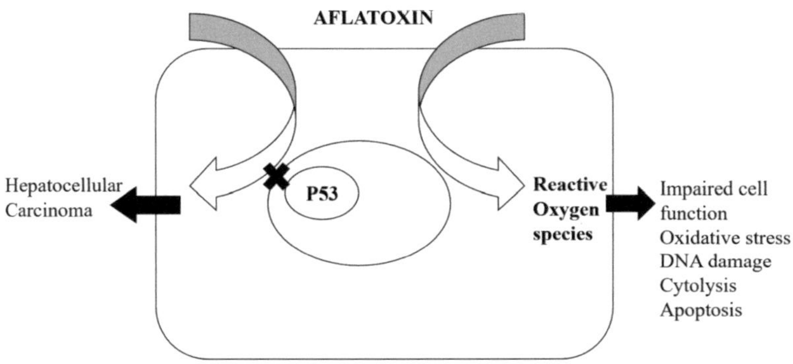

Figure 1.
Mechanism of toxicity of aflatoxin.

childhood cirrhosis (ICC), which is characterized by fatty degeneration of the liver, is also thought to be caused by aflatoxin intoxication [21].

Immunosuppressive effects: AFB1 is toxic to human lymphocytes. The cytotoxicity is responsible for apoptosis, which ultimately leads to lymphopenia. This causes immunosuppression in the host [22].

Effects on reproduction: There are not many studies in this regard, but some researchers reported the toxic effects of aflatoxins on the testis and other reproductive organs. This has harmful consequences on spermatogenesis, which is responsible for decreased sperm count. In one study, it was observed that the disruption of semen parameters was evident in the infertile men having significant levels of aflatoxin in blood and semen as compared to fertile men [23].

3.2 Fumonisins

Fumonisins are a group of mycotoxins mainly produced by various *Fusarium* species. The main sources are *Fusarium verticillioides* (previously, *F. moniliforme*), *F. proliferatum*, *F. nygamai*, and to a lesser extent, other species, such as *F. anthophilum*, *F. dlamini*, *F. napiforme*, *F. subglutinans*, *F. polyphialidicum* and *F. oxysporum* [24]. There are almost 28 types designated as A-series, B-series, C-series, and P-series. The B-series consists of FB1, FB2, and FB3 [1]. *FB1* is the commonest and mainly contaminates *maize or corn* and other foodstuffs such as rice, sorghum, beans, and beer [24].

Fumonisins mainly affect the *sphingolipid biosynthesis* in the hosts. It *inhibits the ceramide synthase* enzyme, which is essential for the conversion of sphinganine and sphingosine to ceramide [25]. Ceramides are the basic structural components of all sphingolipids (found in the cellular membranes of animals and plants) [26]. This results in the accumulation of both sphinganine and sphingosine in the liver and kidneys, resulting in the apoptosis of renal tubule cells and hepatocytes (**Figure 2**) [25].

In humans, fumonisins are associated with *esophageal cancer* and *neural tube defects.* Impairment of sphingolipid biosynthesis, resulting in the disruption of cellular activity, is the key factor in the carcinogenicity of fumonisins in humans [3].

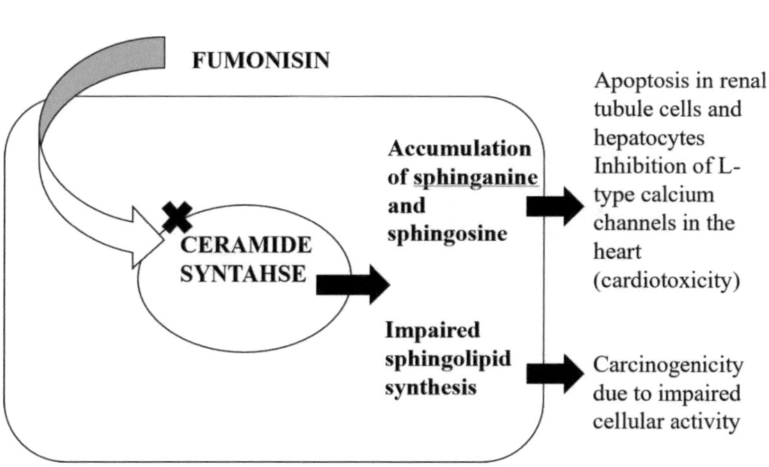

Figure 2.
Mechanism of toxicity of fumonisin.

The IARC classified mycotoxins from *F. verticilloides* as *a Group 2B human carcinogen* [13].

FB1 has a neurotoxic effect in horses, causing *equine leucoencephalomalacia* [27]. It is also responsible for *cardiac insufficiency* in horses exposed to FB1. This is mainly due to the inhibition of L-type calcium channels in the heart, which is caused by the accumulation of sphingosine and sphinganine [25]. In pigs, the target organ is the lungs, which causes *porcine pulmonary edema* [28].

3.3 Trichothecenes

Trichothecenes is a group of cyclic compounds produced as secondary metabolites mostly by fungal species under the genus *Fusarium* and also by species of *Stachybotrys, Trichoderma*, and *Trichothecium*. Among them, *Fusarium trichothecenes* are medically significant and are of great concern in the safety of food and feed safety [29]. There are almost 150 toxins in this group of mycotoxins, but the most significant ones are *deoxynivalenol (DON), nivalenol (NIV), toxin T2, toxin HT2*, and diacetoxyscirpenol (DAS) [30]. DON is the most frequently encountered trichothecene in cereal grains [31]. *F. sporotrichioides* produces mainly T-2 toxin, and *F. graminearum* and *F. culmorum* produce deoxynivalenol, nivalenol, and other related compounds [1].

Trichothecenes are well known for *inhibiting protein synthesis* in eukaryotes by binding to the 60S ribosomal subunit and inhibiting the *peptidyl transferase enzyme*. This results in the cessation of various steps in protein synthesis such as initiation, elongation, and chain termination. This eventually causes inhibition of DNA and RNA synthesis, alteration of cellular membrane structure, mitochondrial dysfunction, and arrest of the cell cycle (**Figure 3**) [32].

The clinical symptoms of trichothecenes intoxication include gastrointestinal such as weight loss, vomiting, feed refusal, diarrhea, hemorrhages, and necrosis of the gastrointestinal epithelium. Trichothecenes also cause significant suppression of immune cells in the thymus, bone marrow, and spleen, causing impaired host immunity. This increases host susceptibility to various opportunistic fungal infections such as candidiasis and cryptococcosis and increases graft rejection in transplant

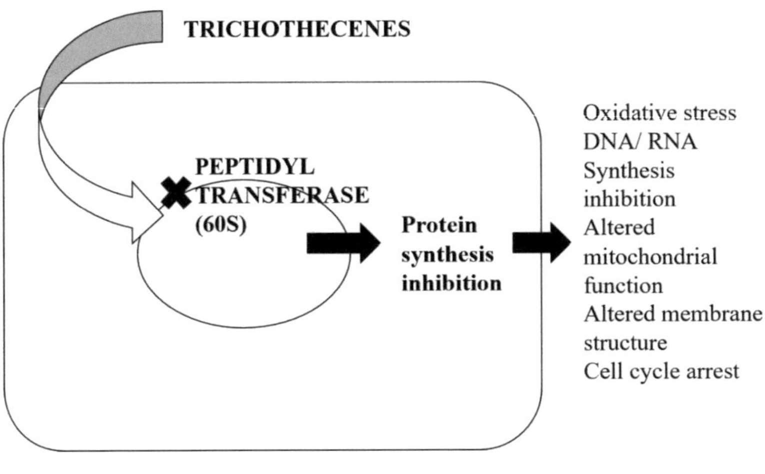

Figure 3.
Mechanism of toxicity of trichothecenes.

recipients. In alimentary toxic aleukia (ATA), the patient presents with gastrointestinal symptoms and leukopenia [1].

3.4 Zearalenone

Zearalenone (ZEN), is also known as *F-2 or RAL mycotoxin*. Chemically, it is similar to estrogen, which is mainly produced by *Fusarium graminearum* and also to some extent by other fungal species under the genus Fusarium such as *F. culmorum, F. cerealis, or F. equiseti* [2].

This toxin is a xenoestrogen, a type of xenohormone that imitates estrogens (sex-steroid hormone mimicry) [33]. It is biochemically identical to natural estrogen in the host, causing estrogenic effects while competing with estrogen receptors, which results in antiestrogenic effects. In females, it causes infertility, vulval edema, vaginal prolapse, and mammary hypertrophy. In males, there are signs of feminization such as testicular atrophy, decreased libido, and enlargement of mammary glands (**Figure 4**) [1].

Estrogen, apart from being a reproductive hormone, has some immune functions. It acts on immune cells with the help of estrogen receptors (ERs) and causes modulation or suppression of immune functions [34]. It also alters the function of the endocrine system by acting as an endocrine-disrupting compound (EDC), potentially leading to adverse health events. They are also known to increase the alterations in physiological functions such as homeostasis, growth, development, and reproduction, which are monitored by sex hormones [35].

3.5 Ochratoxins

Ochratoxins are dihydro-isocoumarins, which can bind to various metabolic byproducts of phenylalanine. They are mainly categorized as ochratoxin A (OTA), B, and C. *Aspergillus ochraceus* is the main source of OTA, and other Aspergillus and Penicillium species (*Penicillium verrucosum*) produces ochratoxin A, B, and C. OTA is the medically significant mycotoxin highly prevalent and responsible for harmful consequences in human health [36]. Ochratoxins are documented to have contaminated various foods like grains, rice, wheat, and dry fruits, as well as beverages like

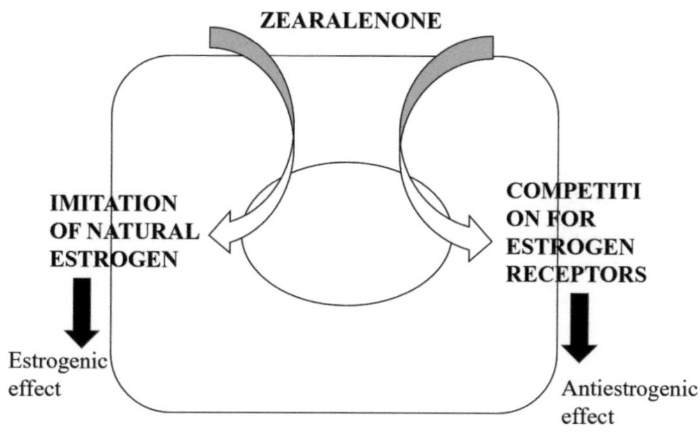

Figure 4.
Mechanism of toxicity of zearalenone.

coffee, wine, and beer. They are fat-soluble and accumulate as a fat depot in animals and while ingested by humans, for example, pork [37].

OTA has the ability to *bind to serum proteins*, for example, *albumin*. This results in decreased renal excretion and accumulation in the target organs [38]. It is also damaging the DNA due to *inhibition of the nuclear factor erythroid 2-related factor 2 (Nrf2)* [39].

OTA is mainly nephrotoxic: They accumulate in kidneys as a result of high vascular flow and tubular re-uptake; hence, they are responsible for renal disorders [1]. In humans, it causes *Balkan endemic nephropathy (BEN)* [40], *chronic interstitial nephropathy (CIN)* [41], renal failure, and tumors [42]. In pigs, it causes *endemic porcine nephropathy* [43].

It is now designated as a *Group 2B possible human carcinogen* due to its carcinogenic properties [13].

3.6 Ergot alkaloids

Ergot alkaloids are mainly produced by *Calviceps purpurea*. The toxic effects result from the consumption of bread made from flours of millet or other grains and rye flours contaminated with Claviceps. The fungus converts the infected grain into a purple, hard, and curved body known as sclerotium. *Ergot is the common name for this sclerotia* [1, 7].

The intoxication occurring due to these alkaloids is called *ergotism*. The ergot alkaloids have *α-adrenergic blocking properties,* which inhibit the response to epinephrine and 5-hydroxy-tryptamine. Ergotism exists in two forms: *gangrenous and convulsive*. In the gangrenous type, there is marked peripheral vasoconstriction and decreased blood circulation, resulting in cold extremities and a burning sensation due to ischemia. This ultimately results in necrosis and gangrene [44].

Ergot alkaloids are also useful in therapeutics due to their unique mechanism of action. These are produced in culture by strains of *Claviceps fusiformis* and *C. paspalum.* They exist in two forms: *ergometrine* (amine alkaloid) and *ergotamine* (amino acid alkaloid). Ergometrine is used clinically due to its *oxytocic effects,* and ergometrine is used in *the treatment of migraine* due to its α-adrenergic blocking and vasoconstriction properties [1, 7].

3.7 Cyclopiazonic acid

It is chemically *indole tetramic acid, derived from tryptophane*, and is related to ergoline alkaloids. It was originally produced by *Penicillium aurantiogriseum* and subsequently by *Penicillium griseofulvum, P. camemberti, P. commune, Aspergillus flavus, A. tamarii, A. oryzae* and *A. versicolor* [1].

It is a *specific inhibitor of ATPase in the intracellular calcium storage sites.* The clinical symptoms start with vomiting, diarrhea, and dehydration, which leads to decreased appetite, loss of weight, and weakness. In severe cases, it may cause depression, opisthotonus, convulsions, and death [1]. In several regions of India, poor people consume kodo millet seeds of rice grass (*Paspalum scrobiculatum*) as a staple food. Ingestion of contaminated seeds causes giddiness, sleepiness, and tremors, which is known as *Kodua poisoning* [45].

3.8 Patulin

Patulin was first derived from *Penicillium patulum* (*P. griseofulvum*) in 1943. Now it is derived from other molds such as *Penicillium, Aspergillus, Paecilomyces*, and *Byssochlamys*. It mainly contaminates apples and apple-derived products and other fruits such as cherries, blueberries, plums, bananas, strawberries, and grapes. The exact mechanism of toxicity is not known but they may cause immunological, neurological, and gastrointestinal symptoms [1, 46].

4. Impact of mycotoxins on gut health and microbiota

Now it is well documented that a healthy gut microbiota is a key factor for the overall health of the host. The gut microbiota has the ability to eliminate mycotoxins from the host's gastrointestinal tract naturally if the host is healthy and has a balanced gut microbiota. Moreover, it is observed that the mycotoxins have the ability to change the composition of gut microbiota. This may result in the elimination of beneficial bacteria and the elevation of gut pathogens [47].

The interactions between gut microbiota and mycotoxins have a significant role in the development of mycotoxicosis, particularly hepatocellular carcinoma (HCC). Gut microbiota perturbation is found to be one of the factors influencing mycotoxin-induced HCC. The development of HCC in mice induced by a combination of diethylnitrosamine (DEN) and hepatotoxin carbon tetrachloride (CCl4) is prevented via gut sterilization [48]. Some specific bacterial species are also found to be correlated with HCC development. Studies demonstrated that in patients of HCC with intestinal colonization by *Helicobacter hepaticus*, the DNA of *Helicobacter* ssp. was only present in liver biopsies from HCC patients, not in control samples [49]. Findings from both animal and human studies demonstrated that liver cirrhosis and HCC stimulate intestinal dysbiosis as well as a significant increase in the population of the *Escherichia coli* and *Atopobium* cluster, coupled with a significant ($P < 0.05$) reduction in the percentages of beneficial microbes such as *Lactobacillus* group, *Bifidobacterium* group, and *Enterococcus* group [50]. A probiotic supplement is an effective dietary approach to decrease the risk of liver cancer, as it reduces the biologically available effective toxic dose of mycotoxin along with the normalization of gut microbiota [47].

5. Emerging mycotoxins

Emerging mycotoxins were defined as "*mycotoxins having increased incidence of toxicity but presently they are not routinely determined and not legislatively regulated*" [51].

According to this definition, many fungal metabolites with toxicity would fall in this category of emerging mycotoxins. The following are the mycotoxins with emerging potential [52]:

5.1 Fusarium metabolites

Enniatins (ENNs), Beauvericin (BEA), Moniliformin (MON), Fusaproliferin (FP), Fusaric acid (FA), Culmorin (CUL), and Butenolide (BUT).

5.2 Aspergillus metabolites

Sterigmatocystin (STE) and Emodin (EMO).

5.3 Penicillium metabolites

Mycophenolic acid (MPA).

5.4 Alternaria metabolites

Alternariol (AOH), Alternariol monomethyl ether (AME), and tenuazonic acid (TeA).

6. Conclusion

Mycotoxins are highly toxic and unavoidable food contaminants that exert serious threats to human and animal health. The common mycotoxins that cause mycotoxicoses quite often are aflatoxins, deoxynivalenol, ochratoxins, zearalenone, and fumonisins. These are produced by various fungal species belonging to the genus *Penicillium, Aspergillus,* and *Fusarium* spp. These fungal species infect many cereals and nut crops and contaminate them with mycotoxin production. The harmful consequences caused by these mycotoxins to human and animal health are immunotoxicity, hepatotoxicity, nephrotoxicity, carcinogenicity, and teratogenicity. One health approach is necessary for the prevention and control of mycotoxicoses.

Author details

Girish Patil*, Archana Keche and Madhavi Madkey
Microbiology Department, All India Institute of Medical Sciences, Raipur, India

*Address all correspondence to: dr.girishpatil2408@gmail.com

References

[1] Chander J. Mycotoxicosis and mycetismus. In: Textbook of Medical Mycology. 4th ed. New Delhi: Jaypee Brothers Medical Publishers; 2018. pp. 772-779

[2] Taheur FB, Fedhila K, Chaieb K, Kouidhi B, Bakhrouf A, Abrunhosa L. Adsorption of aflatoxin B1, zearalenone and ochratoxin a by microorganisms isolated from kefir grains. International Journal of Food Microbiology. 2017;**251**:1-7. DOI: 10.1016/j.ijfoodmicro.2017.03.021

[3] Bezerra E, da Rocha M, Freire FdCO, Erlan Feitosa Maia F, Izabel Florindo Guedes M, Rondina D. Mycotoxins and their effects on human and animal health. Food Control. 2014;**36**:159-165. DOI: 10.1016/j.foodcont.2013.08.021

[4] Rogowska A, Pomastowski P, Sagandykova G, Buszewski B. Zearalenone and its metabolites: Effect on human health, metabolism and neutralization methods. Toxicon. 2019;**162**:46-56. DOI: 10.1016/j.toxicon.2019.03.004

[5] Woolf A. Witchcraft or mycotoxin? The Salem witch trials. Journal of Toxicology. Clinical Toxicology. 2000;**38**(4):457-460. DOI: 10.1081/clt-100100958

[6] Krishnamachari KA, Bhat RV, Nagarajan V, Tilak TB. Hepatitis due to aflatoxicosis. An outbreak in Western India. Lancet. 1975;**1**(7915):1061-1063. DOI: 10.1016/s0140-6736(75)91829-2

[7] Crews C. Analysis of ergot alkaloids. Toxins (Basel). 2015;**7**(6):2024-2050. DOI: 10.3390/toxins7062024

[8] Ngindu A, Johnson BK, Kenya PR, et al. Outbreak of acute hepatitis caused by aflatoxin poisoning in Kenya. Lancet. 1982;**1**:1346-1348. DOI: 10.1016/S0140-6736(82)92411-4

[9] Bhat RV, Beedu SR, Ramakrishna Y, Munshi KL. Outbreak of trichothecene mycotoxicosis associated with consumption of mould-damaged wheat production in Kashmir Valley, India. Lancet. 1989;**1**(8628):35-37. DOI: 10.1016/s0140-6736(89)91684-x

[10] Lye MS, Ghazali AA, Mohan J, et al. An outbreak of acute hepatic encephalopathy due to severe aflatoxicosis in Malaysia. The American Journal of Tropical Medicine and Hygiene. 1995;**53**:68-72

[11] Bhat RV, Shetty PH, Amruth RP, Sudershan RV. A foodborne disease outbreak due to the consumption of moldy sorghum and maize containing fumonisin mycotoxins. Journal of Toxicology. Clinical Toxicology. 1997;**35**(3):249-255. DOI: 10.3109/15563659709001208

[12] Azziz-Baumgartner E, Lindblade K, Gieseker K, et al. Case-control study of an acute aflatoxicosis outbreak, Kenya, 2004. Environmental Health Perspectives. 2005;**113**:1779-1783. DOI: 10.1289/ehp.8384

[13] Ostry V, Malir F, Toman J, Grosse Y. Mycotoxins as human carcinogens-the IARC monographs classification. Mycotoxin Research. 2017;**33**(1):65-73. DOI: 10.1007/s12550-016-0265-7

[14] Kew MC. Aflatoxins as a cause of hepatocellular carcinoma. Journal of Gastrointestinal and Liver Diseases. 2013;**22**(3):305-310

[15] Patriarca A, Pinto VF. Prevalence of mycotoxins in foods and

decontamination. Current Opinion in Food Science. 2017;**14**:50-60. DOI: 10.1016/j.cofs.2017.01.011

[16] Varga J, Frisvad JC, Samson RA. Two new aflatoxin producing species, and an overview of aspergillus section flavi. Studies in Mycology. 2011;**69**(1):57-80. DOI: 10.3114/sim.2011.69.05

[17] Dhanasekaran D, Shanmugapriya S, Thajuddin N, Panneerselvam A. Aflatoxins and aflatoxicosis in human and animals. Aflatoxins-Biochemistry and Molecular Biology. 2011;**10**:221-254. DOI: 10.5772/22717

[18] Doi AM, Patterson PE, Gallagher EP. Variability in aflatoxin B(1)-macromolecular binding and relationship to biotransformation enzyme expression in human prenatal and adult liver. Toxicology and Applied Pharmacology. 2002;**181**(1):48-59. DOI: 10.1006/taap.2002.9399

[19] Asim M, Sarma MP, Thayumanavan L, Kar P. Role of aflatoxin B1 as a risk for primary liver cancer in North Indian population. Clinical Biochemistry. 2011;**44**(14-15):1235-1240. DOI: 10.1016/j.clinbiochem.2011.07.017

[20] Bosetti C, Turati F, La Vecchia C. Hepatocellular carcinoma epidemiology. Best Practice and Research. Clinical Gastroenterology. 2014;**28**(5):753-770. DOI: 10.1016/j.bpg.2014.08.007

[21] Yadgiri B, Reddy V, Tulpule PG, Srikantia SG, Gopalan C. Aflatoxin and Indian childhood cirrhosis. The American Journal of Clinical Nutrition. 1970;**23**(1):94-98. DOI: 10.1093/ajcn/23.1.94

[22] Al-Hammadi S, Marzouqi F, Al-Mansouri A, Shahin A, Al-Shamsi M, Mensah-Brown E, et al. The cytotoxicity of aflatoxin b1 in human lymphocytes. Sultan Qaboos University Medical Journal. 2014;**14**(1):e65-e71. DOI: 10.12816/0003338

[23] Uriah N, Ibeh IN, Oluwafemi F. A study on the impact of aflatoxin on human reproduction. African Journal of Reproductive Health. 2001;**5**(1):106-110. DOI: 10.2307/3583204

[24] Scott PM. Recent research on fumonisins: A review. Food Additives and Contaminants. Part A, Chemistry, Analysis, Control, Exposure and Risk Assessment. 2012;**29**(2):242-248. DOI: 10.1080/19440049.2010.546000

[25] Voss KA, Riley RT. Fumonisin toxicity and mechanism of action: Overview and current perspectives. Food Safety. 2013;**1**(1):2013006. DOI: 10.14252/foodsafetyfscj.2013006

[26] Engelking LR. Chapter 59—Sphingolipids. In: Engelking LR, editor. Textbook of Veterinary Physiological Chemistry. 3rd ed. Boston: Academic Press; 2015. pp. 378-383

[27] Vendruscolo CP, Frias NC, de Carvalho CB, de Sá LR, Belli CB, Baccarin RY. Leukoencephalomalacia outbreak in horses due to consumption of contaminated Hay. Journal of Veterinary Internal Medicine. 2016;**30**(6):1879-1881. DOI: 10.1111/jvim.14588

[28] Freitas B, Mota M, Del Santo T, Afonso E, Silva C, Utimi N, et al. Mycotoxicosis in swine: A review. Journal of Animal Production Advances. 2012;**2**:174-181

[29] Proctor RH, McCormick SP, Kim HS, Cardoza RE, Stanley AM, Lindo L, et al. Evolution of structural diversity of trichothecenes, a family of toxins produced by plant pathogenic and entomopathogenic fungi. PLoS Pathogens. 2018;**14**(4):e1006946. DOI: 10.1371/journal.ppat.1006946

[30] Yang X, Lv Y, Huang K, Luo Y, Xu W. Zinc inhibits aflatoxin B1-induced cytotoxicity and genotoxicity in human hepatocytes (HepG2 cells). Food and Chemical Toxicology. 2016;**92**:17-25. DOI: 10.1016/j.fct.2016.03.012

[31] Tian Y, Tan Y, Liu N, Liao Y, Sun C, Wang S, et al. Functional agents to biologically control deoxynivalenol contamination in cereal grains. Frontiers in Microbiology. 2016;7:395. DOI: 10.3389/fmicb.2016.00395

[32] Arunachalam C, Doohan FM. Trichothecene toxicity in eukaryotes: Cellular and molecular mechanisms in plants and animals. Toxicology Letters. 2013;**217**(2):149-158. DOI: 10.1016/j.toxlet.2012.12.003

[33] Zahran E, Elbahnaswy S, Mamdouh Z, El-Matbouli M. Xenosteroids in aquaculture with special consideration to Lake Manzala (Northern Delta Lake, Egypt): Types, sources and mechanism of action. Aquaculture Research. 2021;**52**:1-16. DOI: 10.1111/are.15504

[34] Islam MR, Kim JW, Roh YS, Kim JH, Han KM, Kwon HJ, et al. Evaluation of immunomodulatory effects of zearalenone in mice. Journal of Immunotoxicology. 2017;**14**(1):125-136. DOI: 10.1080/1547691X.2017.1340371

[35] Kar S, Sangem P, Anusha N, Senthilkumaran B. Endocrine disruptors in teleosts: Evaluating environmental risks and biomarkers. Aquaculture and Fisheries. 2021;**6**:1-26

[36] Marroquín-Cardona AG, Johnson NM, Phillips TD, Hayes AW. Mycotoxins in a changing global environment—A review. Food and Chemical Toxicology. 2014;**69**:220-230. DOI: 10.1016/j.fct.2014.04.025

[37] Kumar P, Mahato DK, Gupta A, Pandey S, Paul V, Saurabh V, et al. Nivalenol mycotoxin concerns in foods: An overview on occurrence, impact on human and animal health and its detection and management strategies. Toxins (Basel). 2022;**14**(8):527. DOI: 10.3390/toxins14080527

[38] Duarte SC, Lino CM, Pena A. Food safety implications of ochratoxin A in animal-derived food products. Veterinary Journal. 2012;**192**(3):286-292. DOI: 10.1016/j.tvjl.2011.11.002

[39] Limonciel A, Jennings P. A review of the evidence that ochratoxin A is an Nrf2 inhibitor: Implications for nephrotoxicity and renal carcinogenicity. Toxins (Basel). 2014;**6**(1):371-379. DOI: 10.3390/toxins6010371

[40] Stiborová M, Arlt VM, Schmeiser HH. Balkan endemic nephropathy: An update on its aetiology. Archives of Toxicology. 2016;**90**(11):2595-2615. DOI: 10.1007/s00204-016-1819-3

[41] Hassen W, Abid S, Achour A, Creppy E, Bacha H. Ochratoxin A and beta2-microglobulinuria in healthy individuals and in chronic interstitial nephropathy patients in the Centre of Tunisia: A hot spot of ochratoxin A exposure. Toxicology. 2004;**199**(2-3):185-193. DOI: 10.1016/j.tox.2004.02.027

[42] Hope JH, Hope BE. A review of the diagnosis and treatment of ochratoxin A inhalational exposure associated with human illness and kidney disease including focal segmental glomerulosclerosis. Journal of Environmental and Public Health. 2012;**2012**:835059. DOI: 10.1155/2012/835059

[43] Jørgensen K, Petersen A. Content of ochratoxin A in paired kidney and meat samples from healthy Danish slaughter pigs. Food Additives and

Contaminants. 2002;**19**(6):562-567. DOI: 10.1080/02652030110113807

[44] Belser-Ehrlich S, Harper A, Hussey J, Hallock R. Human and cattle ergotism since 1900: Symptoms, outbreaks, and regulations. Toxicology and Industrial Health. 2013;**29**(4):307-316. DOI: 10.1177/0748233711432570

[45] Lalitha Rao B, Husain A. Presence of cyclopiazonic acid in kodo millet (*Paspalum scrobiculatum*) causing 'kodua poisoning' in man and its production by associated fungi. Mycopathologia. 1985;**89**(3):177-180. DOI: 10.1007/BF00447028

[46] Channaiah LH. An overview of mycotoxicosis and human's health concerns: A mini-review. Novel Techniques in Nutrition and Food Science. 2019;**4**(1):469-472. DOI: 10.31031/NTNF.2019.04.000576

[47] Liew WP, Mohd-Redzwan S. Mycotoxin: Its impact on gut health and microbiota. Frontiers in Cellular and Infection Microbiology. 2018;**8**:60. DOI: 10.3389/fcimb.2018.00060

[48] Dapito DH, Mencin A, Gwak GY, Pradere JP, Jang MK, Mederacke I, et al. Promotion of hepatocellular carcinoma by the intestinal microbiota and TLR4. Cancer Cell. 2012;**21**(4):504-516. DOI: 10.1016/j.ccr.2012.02.007

[49] Gargano LM, Hughes JM. Microbial origins of chronic diseases. Annual Review of Public Health. 2014;**35**:65-82. DOI: 10.1146/annurev-publhealth-032013-182426

[50] Zhang HL, Yu LX, Yang W, Tang L, Lin Y, Wu H, et al. Profound impact of gut homeostasis on chemically-induced pro-tumorigenic inflammation and hepatocarcinogenesis in rats. Journal of Hepatology. 2012;**57**(4):803-812. DOI: 10.1016/j.jhep.2012.06.011

[51] Vaclavikova M, Malachova A, Veprikova Z, Dzuman Z, Zachariasova M, Hajslova J. 'Emerging' mycotoxins in cereals processing chains: Changes of enniatins during beer and bread making. Food Chemistry. 2013;**136**(2):750-757. DOI: 10.1016/j.foodchem.2012.08.031

[52] Gruber-Dorninger C, Novak B, Nagl V, Berthiller F. Emerging mycotoxins: Beyond traditionally determined food contaminants. Journal of Agricultural and Food Chemistry. 2017;**65**(33):7052-7070. DOI: 10.1021/acs.jafc.6b03413

Chapter 7

Mycotoxins in Chicken Farming: What You Need to Know

Fabrice De Paul Tatfo Keutchatang, Isabelle Sandrine Bouelet Ntsama and Paul Richard Keutchatang

Abstract

Poultry farming is an activity that is booming all over the world. Unfortunately, the sector can be attacked by mycotoxins that could be the cause of a wide range of damage, including mycotoxicosis, which are diseases that have negative effects on the welfare of chickens and therefore on the profitability of the poultry sector. The main aim of this chapter is to raise awareness of the issues surrounding mycotoxins in poultry farming. Therefore, data of a literature search were collected and a survey in a number of farms was conducted. As a result, farmers surveyed are not awarded about biosecurity measures and good practices in poultry. These have several consequences as frequent diseases, death of birds, and discouragement of farmers. There is lack of document for small farmers, reason why they are not awarded about the existence of molds as well as mycotoxins leading to side effects. The decreasing of side effects of these consequences goes through the respect of good poultry practices, biosecurity measures, and the permanent control of the safety quality of feed ingredients.

Keywords: poultry, mycotoxins, molds, biosecurity measure, Cameroon

1. Introduction

Poultry farming is the rearing of poultry, particularly chickens as main group. It is an activity that is booming all over the world. Cameroon is no exception to this vast movement in the poultry sector [1]. What is more, its position on the African continent, more specifically in Central Africa; its climatic diversity; and the dynamism of its population make it a veritable Africa of beauty, a major production basin for chickens and eggs [1]. However, this climatic diversity could be a brake on exponential growth in the poultry sector because of the microscopic fungi responsible for the production of mycotoxins. Mycotoxins are biologically active toxic secondary metabolites produced by toxigenic fungi that invade crops in the field. These toxigenic fungi can also grow on food during storage and secrete toxins [2, 3]. These mycotoxins could be the cause of a wide range of damage, including mycotoxicosis, which are diseases that have negative effects on the welfare of chickens and therefore on the profitability of the poultry sector [4, 5]. However, many actors in the poultry sector are still very poorly informed about mycotoxins and the various issues involved in the poultry sector. The main aim of this chapter is to raise awareness of the issues surrounding mycotoxins in poultry farming. The data contained in this chapter are the result of a literature search and a survey in a number of farms.

2. General information on mycotoxins in chicken farming

2.1 Origin

Mycotoxins are produced by toxigenic fungi, mainly belonging to the *Aspergillus*, *Fusarium* and *Penicillium* species, which invade crops in the field [6]. Fungi are eukaryotic microorganisms with cells comprising a nucleus, cytoplasm, and cytoplasmic membrane. There are several types of fungi, including toxigenic fungi or molds capable of secreting dangerous toxins under certain conditions [6]. The toxins secreted by toxigenic fungi are numerous and vary depending on the sector of activity. In poultry farming, the toxins frequently encountered and studied are aflatoxins (AF), citrinins (CIT), fumonisins (F), ochratoxins (OT), and tricothecenes. These toxins mainly come from chicken feed, which is a mixture of several inputs or ingredients that make feed important substrates for the growth of toxin-secreting molds [7–10].

2.2 Condition for mold growth and mycotoxin production

These are factors that encourage the development of molds, which in turn secrete mycotoxins or toxins. In the poultry sector, these factors include [7–11]:

- The nature and quality of the hen house or building: the construction of the hen house must comply with certain standards, such as its position or direction, which must be parallel to the direction of the wind, its height, the quality of the materials used, ventilation, and insulation of the roof. When construction standards are not respected, as is the case with many small-scale chicken farmers, molds can develop and secrete toxins that end up in the farming environment.

- Where feeds are stored: feeds should be stored in ventilated areas where relative humidity is low. Food is a mixture of several inputs, the majority of which are cereals, which are good growth substrates for molds. This means that when feed is stored in dark, unventilated rooms with high relative humidity, as is the case with many small-scale chicken farmers, the feed not only sweats but also absorbs water. As a result, the water content of feed increases, making it highly available and, along with other nutrients such as the carbohydrates present in feed, encouraging the development of molds and therefore the secretion of mycotoxins.

- The temperature in the hen house during rearing: the temperature in the hen house during rearing is a crucial factor that seems to be neglected by many poultry farmers and chicken breeders. As the temperature rises, relative humidity falls and vice versa. This means that the temperature in the henhouse must be neither too low nor too high. If the temperature is too low, the humidity will rise and the litter or feed will become too damp, conditions that are favorable to the growth of molds.

- The maturity and degree of drying of inputs such as maize: some ingredients, such as maize, have a high-water content, which is all the more important when the maize is not yet fully mature. When inputs, especially maize in our context, are not fully matured and less dry, they are a good substrate for mold growth and development, both on their own and in combination with other inputs. As a result, a feed formulated with the new maize would have a higher probability of being a good substrate for mold development, unlike the old maize, which, because of the length of time it took, would have had time to dry well, with the advantage of a much lower water content.

- The length of time the feed remains in the feeding troughs: the longer the feed remains in the troughs, the greater the substrate is for mold growth and development.

- The level at which the drinking troughs are filled: if the troughs are too full, especially if they are not automatic, the water can spill out when you turn them over, wetting the bedding and feed, which then become important areas for the growth and development of mold.

- The length of time the feed is stored: if the feed spends a lot of time in the henhouse or inside the henhouse, this is not very advisable, as the longer the feed is stored, the more likely it is to absorb water and become very damp, thus favoring the growth of molds and the secretion of mycotoxins or toxins.

- The origin of inputs or ingredients could be a factor favoring mold growth: depending on the agroecological zone, the chemical composition of the various ingredients and therefore their water content may vary. This means that if the water content of an ingredient is high, the feed is more likely to be a good substrate for mold growth and development, especially when it is known that the frequency of contamination of raw materials or ingredients is often between 30% and 70%. This frequency of contamination can sometimes be even higher for certain raw material/toxin combinations.

2.3 Behavior of mycotoxins in chickens

Once in the chicken's body, mycotoxins can accumulate in tissues or organs such as the liver and cause mycotoxicosis, as well as many other harmful effects. Mycotoxins undergo a series of transformations including absorption, distribution, metabolism, and excretion or elimination (**Figure 1**) [12–14].

- *Absorption*: Absorption corresponds to the phase of dissolution and appearance of the active ingredients in the blood, involving transmembrane passage.

- *Distribution*: After absorption, the mycotoxins are transported in the blood through circulation, carrying them to the various organs and tissues: this is the distribution phase.

- *Biotransformations or metabolism*: Metabolism is one of the most important factors affecting the overall toxic profile of a mycotoxin. The biotransformation or

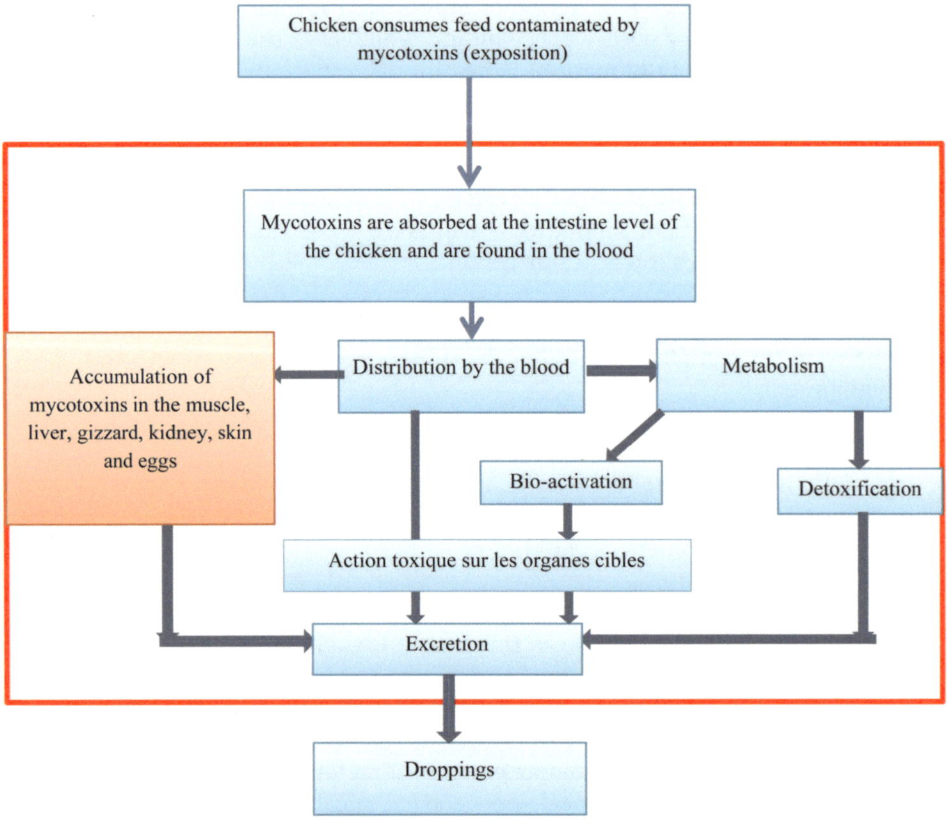

Figure 1.
Behavior of mycotoxins once in the chicken body.

metabolic reactions undergone by mycotoxins can lead to detoxification either by inactivation, that is, chemical blocking of the groups responsible for the toxic activity, or by an increase in water solubility by glucuro-conjugation, favoring fecal elimination.

Figure 1 shows schematically how mycotoxins behave once in the chicken body.

3. Some elements affected by mycotoxins

Many elements are affected by mycotoxins once they enter the animal body. These include [12–16]:

- The kidney: kidney is an important excretory and purifying organ. When it is affected by toxins such as aflatoxins, patulin, and ochratoxin A, this leads to numerous dysfunctions that affect the entire animal organism. The kidney is also an important organ of excretion and purification.

- The genes: genes are the portion of DNA that govern the synthesis of a protein. The toxic effect of certain toxins on genes could lead to abnormal proteins and therefore inactive enzymes unable to play their role properly. When enzymes are inactive or proteins are abnormal, this can have an impact on the animal's metabolism and lead to stunted growth.

- The immune system is the body's defense system: when it is affected or disrupted, this can have a number of consequences, such as the persistence of disease, immunomodulation, and permanent stress in chickens.
- The red blood: red blood cells are specialized in transporting respiratory gases and certain nutrients throughout the body. When they are affected or destroyed by certain substances, there is a drop in their numbers in the body and they become unable to carry out their function. As a result, cells can become deprived of oxygen and overloaded with carbon dioxide, leading to respiratory stress, tiredness, and programmed cell death in chickens.
- The central nervous system is the body's command center. When it is damaged, many effects can be seen in chickens, such as loss of balance, impaired vision, and digestive problems due to poor nutrition.
- The reproductive system is the system that enables reproduction and, in the case of layers, egg production. When it is affected by toxins, this represents a danger for the poultry industry, not only because it leads to a drop in egg production but also because of malformations in the eggs, which may also be of poor quality.

4. Practical observations and impacts of mycotoxins on the chicken's well-being and chicken farming

4.1 Practical observations

During a survey of some small broiler and layer farmers (see survey sheet in Appendix A), it was noted that of the 90 farms surveyed, 75 (83.3%) did not have a suitable ventilation system and the feed was kept either in a corner of the farm building or in a hermetically sealed shop to prevent birds and rodents from entering. In such conditions, the feed may find itself sweating and therefore releasing water (sweat). Given that the feed is a mixture of several ingredients of varying nutritional composition, the water released by sweating makes it an excellent substrate for the growth of molds, which in turn secrete toxins or mycotoxins, secondary metabolites found in the feed, making it dangerous for the chicken. Also in our study, samples of feed consumed by adult broilers and active layers were contaminated with total aflatoxins, aflatoxin B_1, and ochratoxin A at levels sometimes exceeding the recommended levels for these toxins in chicken feed [17]. In such circumstances, the feed is not compliant because it is a reservoir of numerous toxins that can have harmful effects on the chickens, leading to animal malaise and numerous losses associated with mortality, poor growth, and a drop in the laying rate for layers [11, 13].

During the survey of farmers, it became clear from consulting the monitoring sheets that some farmers were not laying at a stable rate and that the mortality rate sometimes exceeded the predicted 5%. In addition, growth was not always uniform within the same band, probably due to the high incidence of certain diseases [18]. This could also be due to the fact that some farmers were incorporating the medicines into their feed. In fact, if the feed is already contaminated with mycotoxins and veterinary medicines are incorporated into this feed, this could lead to an antagonistic effect or an opposite effect in favor of the mycotoxins.

In another practical case observed during a 50-day cross-sectional study on a broiler farm, a feed containing mycotoxins was responsible for high mortality during the hot hours of the day. In fact, during this experimental phase, we could see that in the morning, the chickens fed a feed containing no antitoxin were still doing well until around 11.30 am. But between midday and 4 pm, especially when it was sunny, the same feed caused negative behavior or seizures in the chickens, followed by death. These seizures manifested themselves as shallow breathing, followed by agitation, and then, the chicken ended up with its back to the ground and eventually died. On the other hand, when the chickens were fed only water during these hot hours of the day, no crisis was observed and no deaths occurred. Hence, when broilers were fed after 4 pm to 5 pm, no crisis and mortality was not observed.

Aflatoxins analyzed in feed could lead to impaired liver and kidney function, as well as being immunosuppressive. As a result, the absorption of aflatoxins through feed, as observed during the survey, could lead to a deterioration in growth in broilers and, in the case of laying hens, a reduction in egg-laying rate and eggshell quality. Some authors have reported a reduction in the effectiveness of vaccination and an increase in mortality as adverse effects of ingesting aflatoxin-containing feed.

Alongside aflatoxins, ochratoxin A was also present in feed for broilers and layers. This presence poses a danger not only to the welfare of the chickens but also to farmers and even consumers. It has been reported that the kidney is the target organ for ochratoxin A, which is also a hepatotoxic and immunosuppressive toxin. Although less sensitive because of their high excretion capacity, poultry are exposed to many of the negative effects of ochratoxin. Kidney damage, reduced feed intake, delayed growth, reduced egg-laying rates and shell quality, and increased early mortality have all been reported.

4.2 Impacts of mycotoxins on the chicken well-being and chicken poultry

In addition to the mycotoxins already analyzed and their effects reported above, many other toxins can have harmful effects on the well-being of chickens and on chicken farming itself. These include [12–14]:

- T2 mycotoxin: it has been reported that poultry tend to be more sensitive to trichothecenes, such as T2, than other animals such as ruminants. The toxic effects of T2 mycotoxin can be classified as genotoxic and cytotoxic. T2 toxin affects the immune system, the cells of the digestive and hepatic systems, the nervous system, and the skin, causing oral and skin lesions. It can also compromise certain production parameters (growth and egg-laying).

- Deoxynivalenol (DON): it belongs to the group of trichothecenes and is distinguished by its cytotoxic effect, interfering with protein synthesis and damaging DNA after inducing oxidative stress. It has also been reported that DON can be immunosuppressive or immunomodulatory, depending on the concentration ingested, and alter various functions of the intestinal tract by compromising permeability or the absorption surface. The ingestion of DON through food could be the cause of reduced growth, egg-laying rate, and egg quality.

- Fumonisins: Fumonisins are among the most dangerous toxins, on a par with aflatoxins. Among fumonisins, fumonisin B_1 is characterized by the damage it causes to the liver. What is more, after a long period of ingesting feed contaminated with low doses of fumonisins, animals reduce their consumption and growth. Fumonisin is also an immunosuppressive mycotoxin that can impair nerve function. In this context, fumonisin poisoning has also been associated with increased mortality in poultry.

- Zearalenone: Poultry are less affected by zearalenone than other monogastric animals, such as pigs. This difference is due to various factors, including the low absorption and rapid elimination of metabolites produced in the liver of poultry. The effects of zearalenone are mainly on the reproductive system, as it acts like an estrogen hormone. It is also responsible for reductions in egg-laying and egg size, as well as an increase in embryonic mortality. In males, it reduces the percentage of fertilization. However, these cases are observed after ingestion of high doses of zearalenone. Zeralenone is very dangerous in the case of multi-contamination, since it exacerbates the negative effects produced by other mycotoxins, such as aflatoxin B_1 or DON, on production yields, the immune system, the liver, and the intestinal barrier.

4.3 Some techniques for recognizing mycotoxins

They are a number of simple techniques that farmers can use to detect molds and therefore mycotoxins in their inputs or ingredients. These include:

- The color of the ingredient, which involves the eyes: this gives an idea of the quality of the ingredient in relation to the mycotoxins. Generally speaking, ingredients affected by toxins generally have a black color tending toward rottenness. This is particularly true of ingredients such as maize, groundnuts, and soya, which are of poor quality and therefore affected by or containing mycotoxins. Farmers therefore need to be vigilant when they go to have feed manufactured. This is all the more true because many people think that what is bad is destined for the animal, forgetting the principle that what goes in is what comes out, which means that if you give the animal what is bad, it will only produce what is bad and therefore not good for human consumption. However, the mold that secretes mycotoxins can be black, white, or green in color and can take on an orange tinge when it proliferates outside the ingredient.

- The taste that involves the tongue: ingredients affected by mycotoxins generally have a very better taste.

- Behavior in water: when ingredients are immersed in water, those of poor quality usually float, while those of good quality sink. The fact that the input floats does not necessarily mean that it is affected by mycotoxins. It simply means that the input is not of good quality and this poor quality could be due to the presence of mycotoxins.

- The smell that involves the nose: the smell of mold is very strong and permeates the tissues. So, the farmer can take ingredients of different quality in both hands and smell them. Generally speaking, moldy ingredients have a much stronger odor that tends to stifle breathing.

- The behavior of inputs, especially maize, once in the soil: farmers can simply set aside a small area of land on their farm to detect molds or mycotoxins in their maize. To do this, he will need to take a few maize seeds and sow them in a place where there is sufficient water, humus, and a good temperature. After a week, he will notice that the moldy seeds either will not germinate, or will germinate, but the seedlings will be stunted and large, pale yellow in color.

- The behavior of the feed on the farm, its texture, and its smell: when feed is stored on the farm for a long time or in poor conditions, it transpires and expands. As a result, the feed is neither crumbly nor granulated, and its smell is different from that of normal feed. In such circumstances, the feed is moldy and could be dangerous for the chickens.

4.4 Farmers' knowledge of mycotoxins

Farmers' knowledge of mycotoxins and therefore of molds is still rudimentary in the sense that many farmers think that since chickens are animals, they should be given everything that is bad. In fact, during the survey of 90 farmers, around 70 said they knew nothing about molds, let alone mycotoxins. This represents a danger for their business and for the well-being of their birds, because prevention is better than cure. So, the more you know, the more careful you are and the less serious the consequences. As a result, some farmers, especially the smaller ones, find themselves taking moldy maize and groundnuts—in short, anything that is rotten—to make chicken feed. This could be at the root of the large number of deaths caused by mycotoxicosis. This is a danger for poultry farming because many farmers could be discouraged by this ignorance. This discouragement could lead to the cessation of poultry farming and create a food safety problem, given the nutritional and dietary benefits of poultry products such as chicken meat and eggs.

Ignorance of the existence and presence of mycotoxins and molds in the poultry sector could be at the root of conflicts between farmers or between farmers and occupants of the area where the poultry house is located. In one practical case, during a field visit as part of a survey of farmers, we were confronted with a case where the farmer accused the villagers of being witches. The farmer woke up one morning to find around 500 of the 1000 35-day-old broilers on his farm dead. When he was approached, he was furious and said that the villagers, who wanted to eat the chicken, had put poison in the water so that the chickens would die, and that he was giving it to them for free, calling them witches. The whole story had to be pieced together before he realized that the problem was not the water but the feed, because for the last 3 days, he had been feeding the chickens a new feed made from rotten (moldy) maize and groundnut cakes that he had bought well in advance and stored. All he had to do was to change the feed on the same evening to see the mortality drop sharply and cancel itself out with the same water that he had assumed was poisoned. Farmers also need to be made aware of the existence of maximum limits for mycotoxins in feed, even though these are not visible to the naked eye.

4.5 Maximum limits for mycotoxins in chicken feed

In order to limit the negative impact of mycotoxins in the poultry sector, maximum limits for these mycotoxins in chicken feed have been drawn up by international bodies such as the European Commission and the Food and Drug Administration on the basis of scientific studies. Farmers must also be informed of the existence of these limits just for their crop. On the basis of these maximum values, feed can be classified as compliant when the concentration of any mycotoxin in the feed is less than or equal to the value of the maximum limit, and noncompliant when the concentration of the mycotoxin is greater than the value of the maximum limit. In simple terms, when the feed is noncompliant, it is not advisable to use it to feed chickens of any age because of the harmful effects that could lead to discomfort and therefore the death of the chickens. These maximum limits normally vary from one mycotoxin to another, from one age to another, and should also normally vary from one region to another, or even from one country to another. The maximum limits for some mycotoxins according to the organisms mentioned above are shown in **Table 1** [19, 20].

Species	Mycotoxins	Maximum limit recommended (μg/mg, of body weight)	
		EC	FDA
Poultry	Fumonisins (FB_1 + FB_2)	20,000	100,000
Poultry	Deoxynivalenol	5000	10,000
Poultry	Zearalenone	2000	
Poultry	Ochratoxin A	100	
Poultry (without young)	Aflatoxin B_1	10	
Young poultry	Aflatoxin B_1	5	
Poultry	Ergot	1,000,000	
Poultry	T2 + HT2	250	
Young poultry	Total aflatoxins		20
Adult poultry	Total aflatoxins		100
Poultry	Total aflatoxins		300

Table 1.
The maximum limits for some mycotoxins.

4.6 Combating molds practically at the farm level

Practically speaking, to combat mold on farms, farmers must respect certain conditions that are specific to their geographical space, their environment, their locality, and their means. Among these, we can cite:

- Control of the parameters (temperature, relative humidity, ventilation ...) of the storage or storage environment for feeds and medicines;
- Check the nature of the support on which feeds are placed during storage;
- Check the condition of the floor or ground on which the support on which feeds will be placed is placed. Indeed, the floor must be very dry as well as the walls;
- Compliance with hygiene rules and therefore good poultry practices;

- Rigorous control of each ingredient before formulating because if the ingredients are of poor quality and therefore contaminated by mycotoxins, necessarily the final feed obtained will be of poor quality, that is to say, containing mycotoxins;
- Raising awareness among stakeholders in the poultry sector about the existence of mycotoxins and their harmful effects both on their activity and on the health of the consumer;
- Protect the farm or henhouse from wild animals, especially birds, which are vectors of not only germs but also mycotoxins through their secretions such as crusts or droppings.

When formulating feed at the feed mill level, farmers may be advised to prefer old corn to new corn because of its much lower moisture content. Specifically in our context where corn is used as the major ingredient, it is preferable to use old corn, that is to say, that which was harvested before compared to the new one. The old corn is distinguished from the new by the noise (ching for the old and chuack for the new).

We can also cite:

- Control permanently and rigorously the temperature and humidity in the poultry house;
- Avoid feed staying in the feeders for a long time by avoiding putting a lot of feed in the feeders;
- Change water regularly in the drinkers;
- Avoid pouring water on the ground and avoid putting too much water in the drinkers, especially when they are not automatic, at the risk of pouring water onto the litter or feed when turning them over.

In addition to the measures mentioned above, the farmer should take the time to observe the chicks and chickens throughout the day to detect unusual behavior or seizures in the birds and take appropriate action. As a preventive method, we recommend avoiding feeding birds with feed during the hot hours of the day, but rather giving them plenty of fresh water.

5. The economic issues of mycotoxins and molds

Mycotoxins can cause significant economic losses in the poultry sector. Diseases caused by mycotoxins are capable of decimating many chicks or chickens in a short time, and the management of these diseases requires medications that are very expensive, which means that in one way or another, if precautions are not taken, the farmer can find himself losing a lot of chicks or chickens in a flock or spending a lot of money on the purchase drugs in order to save a gang. In the latter case at the end of the band, the cost of producing a chicken or an egg becomes higher than the selling price or even if it is lower than the selling price; the total sale chickens cannot cover the expenses incurred for this band. This leads to discouragement that could be the cause of stopping the poultry activity or reducing the workforce for the most determined. Given that the contribution of the poultry sector to the gross domestic product (GDP) is not negligible, the losses caused by mycotoxins could be at the origin of the reduction in this contribution with the consequence of an overall fall in GDP and therefore poverty.

The main pathways for the synthesis of mycotoxins are: the pentose phosphate pathway, the triose pathway, the amino acid pathway, the polyacetate pathway, and the terpene pathway. These different pathways mostly lead to important intermediates such as acetyl coenzyme A that could be exploited in the poultry industry for useful economic purposes, particularly in metabolism. To do this, studies must be carried out on its different pathways in order to know when its intermediates are produced and how to recover them and use them as additives in chicken feed. These studies require significant funding, and if the results obtained are conclusive, they could generate a lot of financial resources and thereby reduce mortality and therefore losses linked to mycotoxins.

Certain molds are of great importance in improving production yields. Indeed, when the seeds are coated with these molds before being sown, they make it possible to improve certain agronomic parameters such as growth emergence, plant and root length, as well as biomass. In such circumstances, the yield is better and the production good. As a result, the farmer who produces corn intended for poultry farming will have a good production that will be able to feed several flocks at a significant economic cost. In addition, when the seeds are coated with molds recognized as having great agronomic importance, the latter inhibit toxigenic molds (which produce dangerous toxins) and therefore the production of mycotoxins.

6. Conclusion

Mycotoxins in the poultry sector have many consequences. These consequences are visible on the economic level with significant economic losses, on the food security level with nutrient losses linked to significant mortalities, and on the health level with the marketing of poultry products of poor health quality. The decreasing of side effects of these consequences goes through the respect of good poultry practices, biosecurity measures, and the permanent control of the safety quality of feed ingredients. Reducing the harmful effects of these consequences requires compliance with good poultry practices, biosecurity measures, and permanent control of the health quality of feed ingredients. However, the molds responsible for the synthesis of mycotoxins are for certain of a great contribution because they promote better agronomic factors and inhibit the growth of toxigenic molds and therefore the synthesis of mycotoxins. However, mycotoxins are therefore a silent problem in poultry production that must be addressed to reduce their negative effects on poultry health.

Acknowledgements

We acknowledge the cooperation of the chicken farmers who took part in this investigation because they believe that research and collaborations with scientists are an essential step to ensure the quality and safety of products consumed.

Authors' contributions

Fabrice De Paul Tatfo Keutchatang designed the research protocol, collected data, and drafted the chapter under the guidance of Isabelle Sandrine Bouelet Ntsama. All activities were coordinated by Fabrice De Paul Tatfo Keutchatang. Finally, all authors read and approved the final edition of the chapter.

Competing interests

The authors declare that there is no conflict of interest.

Appendix A. Survey sheet or form

Appendice 1 : **Survey sheet or form**

Survey on feed conservation in modern chicken rearing

Date...

Name of the investigator:...

I- Poultry farm identification and information

Town :………………………………………

Location………………………………………

Identification code……………………………

1- What types of poultry do you have on your farm?

Tick the suitable answer

Broilers ☐ Others:…………………………...

Layers ☐

2- Number of building in the farm? ________________

3- Capacity of each building___________________________

4- Number of chickens per building______________________

5- Age of chickens (in weeks)

0-4 ☐ *4-8* ☐ *8-12* ☐ *12-16* ☐

6- What is the source for your chicks?

Certified ☐ Non-certified ☐

Unknown ☐

If is certified source, what are his name and his localization: ___________________________

7- Do you have worker at the farm?

Yes ☐ No ☐

If so, where do they live?

On the premises of the farm ☐

Outside the farm ☐

In the neighborhood of the farm ☐

DOI: http://dx.doi.org/10.5772/intechopen.1006897

II- Quality control

1- What is the administration method of these veterinary drugs?

Water ☐

Feed ☐

Both water and feed ☐

Others……………………………………………………………………

Is there a place where feeds are stored?

Yes ☐ No ☐

If yes which?

Storage room ☐

Poultry house ☐

Others…………………………………………………………….....

2- What is the source of feeds?

Certified commercial ☐

Non-certified commercial ☐

Unknown ☐

3- Does a proper ventilation system exist?

Yes ☐ No ☐

Do you regularly wash the feeding?

Yes ☐ No ☐

4- Are you aware of the existence of molds

Yes ☐ No ☐

5- Do you know about the mycotoxins

Yes ☐ No ☐

If yes how?………………………………………………………………………………………

……………………………………………………………………………………………………

Author details

Fabrice De Paul Tatfo Keutchatang[1,2*], Isabelle Sandrine Bouelet Ntsama[1,3] and Paul Richard Keutchatang[4]

1 Department of Biochemistry, Laboratory for Food Science and Metabolism, Faculty of Sciences, University of Yaoundé 1, Yaoundé, Cameroon

2 Centre for Food and Nutrition Research, IMPM, Yaoundé, Cameroon

3 Advanced Teacher's Training College for Technical Education, University of Douala, Douala, Cameroon

4 DJATAT entreprises, Ndikiniméki, Cameroon

*Address all correspondence to: fabricetatfo@yahoo.fr

References

[1] Teleu Ngandeu E, Ngatchou A. First Assessment of the Poultry Sector in Cameroon: Structure and importance of the commercial and family poultry sector for a better understanding of the issue of Avian Influenza. In: Emergency Assistance for the Control and Prevention of Avian Influenza. National Consultants Report. Food and Agricultural Organization, Project OSRO/GLO/MUL. Yaoundé, Cameroon: FAO Representation; 2006. pp. 1-46. Available from: http://www.fao.org/docs/eims/upload/213743/agal_poultrysector_cameroun_may06_fr.pdf

[2] Gauthier A. Les mycotoxines dans l'alimentation et leur incidence sur la santé. Sciences Pharmaceutiques. 2016. ffdumas-01315198f

[3] Aldridge DC, Turner WB. Fungal Metabolites II. London, New-York: Academic Press; 1983. 631 p

[4] Adetunji MC, Alika OP, Awa NP, Atanda OO, Mwanza M. Microbiological quality and risk assessment for aflatoxins in groundnuts and roasted cashew nuts meant for human consumption. Journal of Toxicology. 2018, 2018. 11 pages. DOI: 10.1155/2018/1308748

[5] Austwick PKC, Aflatoxicosis in Poultry. In: Wyllie TD, Morehouse LG, editors. Mycotoxic Fungi, Mycotoxins, Mycotoxicosis; an encyclopedic handbook. Vol. 2. Mercel Dekker, New York: Mycotoxicosis of Domestic and Laboratory Animals, Poultry and Aquatic Invertebrates and Vertebrates. 1978. pp. 279-301

[6] Zinedine A, Manes J. Occurrence and legislation of mycotoxins in food and feed from Morrocco. Food Control. 2009;**20**:334-344

[7] Abia WA, Simo GN, Warth B, Suyolk M, Krska R, Tchana A, et al. Determination of multiple mycotoxins levels in poultry feeds from Cameroon. Japanese Journal of Veterinary Research. 2013a;**61**(Suppl):S33-S39. Available from: http://hdl.handle.net/2115/52353/10.14943/jjvr.61.suppl.s33

[8] Akinmusire OO, El-Yuguda AD, Musa JA, Oyedele OA, Sulyok M, Somorin YM, et al. Mycotoxins in poultry feed and feed ingredients in Nigeria. Mycotoxin Research. 2018; **35**(2):149-155. DOI: 10.1007/s12550-018-0337-y

[9] Mokubedi SM, Phoku JZ, Changwa RN, Gbashi SPB. Analysis of mycotoxins contamination in poultry feeds manufactured in selected provinces of South Africa using UHPLG-MS/MS. Toxins. 2019;**11**(8):452. DOI: 10.3390/toxins11080452

[10] Hohler D. Ochratoxin A in food and feed: Occurrence, legislation and mode of action. Zeitschrift für Ernährungswissenschaft. 1998;**37**:2-12

[11] Pfohl-Leszkowicz A. Les Mycotoxines Dans L'alimentation: Évaluation et Gestion du Risque. Paris: Tec&Doc; 1999. 478 p

[12] Agence Française de Sécurité Sanitaire des Aliments AFSSA. Évaluation des Risques liés à la Présence de Mycotoxines Dans les Chaînes Alimentaires Humaine et Animale. Rapport Final. French Agency for Food Safety AFSSA. Risk Assessment of Mycotoxins in the Food and Feed Chains. Final Report. Maison Alfort; 2009. 308 p

[13] Zain ME. Impact of mycotoxins on humans and animals. Journal of Saudi Chemical Society. 2011;**15**(2):129-144

[14] Inger V, Eva S-M, Czerny C-P. The carry-over of mycotoxins in products of animal origin with special regard to its implications for the European Food Safety Legislatio. Food and Nutrition Sciences. 2011;**2**:852-867

[15] Food and Agricultural Organization (FAO). Poultry Development Review. 2013. 127 p. ISBN: 978-92-5-108067-2 (PDF). Available from: https://www.fao.org/3/i3531e/i3531e.pdf

[16] Hussain Z, Khan MZ, Khan A, Javed I, Saleemi MK, Mahmood S, et al. Residues of aflatoxinB1 in broiler meat: Effect of age and dietary aflatoxin B1 levels. Food and Chemical Toxicology. 2010;**48**:3304-3307

[17] Keutchatang FDPT, Mafogang B, Kamgain ADT, Nguegwouo E, Tene HM, Ntsama ISB, at al. Mycotoxins and Heavy Metals of Poultry Feeds from the Centre, Littoral, and Western Regions of Cameroon. Journal of World's Poultry Research. 2023;**13**(1):81-88. DOI: 10.36380/jwpr.2023.8

[18] Gondam M, Tatfo Keutchatang F, Yangoua Mafo H, Kansci G, Medoua Nama G. Antimicrobial usage in the chicken farming in Yaoundé, Cameroon: A cross-sectional study. International Journal of Food Contamination. 2016;**3**: 10. DOI: 10.1186/s40550-016-0034-6

[19] Commission Européenne (CE). Règlement (UE) n° 37/2010 de la Commission du 22 décembre 2009 relatif aux substances pharmacologiquement actives et à leur classification en ce qui concerne les limites maximales de résidus dans les aliments d'origine animale. Journal Officiel de l'Union Européenne. 2010;**L 15**:1-72

[20] United States Food and Drug Administration (USFDA). Guidance for Industry: Action Levels for Poisonous or Deleterious Substances in Human Food and Animal Feed. Silver Spring, MD, USA: United States Food and Drug Administration; 2000